Veterinary Genetics and Reproductive Physiology

To Wyn and Reg

For Elsevier:

Commissioning Editor: Mary Seager
Development Editor: Rebecca Nelemans
Project Manager: Joannah Duncan
Designer: Andy Chapman
Illustration Manager: Bruce Hogarth
Illustrator: Jane Fallows

Veterinary Genetics and Reproductive Physiology

By Susan Long BVMS PhD DECAR MRCVS

Referral Consultant for canine reproduction
Academic Advisor, Napier University
Visiting Senior Lecturer, University of Bristol

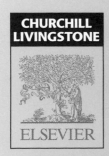

CHURCHILL LIVINGSTONE

ELSEVIER

Edinburgh   London   New York   Oxford   Philadelphia   St Louis   Sydney   Toronto   2006

**BUTTERWORTH
HEINEMANN**
ELSEVIER

First published 2006

ISBN 0 7506 8877 7

British Library Cataloguing in Publication Data
A catalogue record for this book is available from the British Library

Library of Congress Cataloging in Publication Data
A catalog record for this book is available from the Library of Congress

Knowledge and best practice in this field are constantly changing. As new
research and experience broaden our knowledge, changes in practice,
treatment and drug therapy may become necessary or appropriate. Readers
are advised to check the most current information provided (i) on procedures
featured or (ii) by the manufacturer of each product to be administered, to
verify the recommended dose or formula, the method and duration of
administration, and contraindications. It is the responsibility of the
practitioner, relying on their own experience and knowledge of the patient,
to make diagnoses, to determine dosages and the best treatment for each
individual patient, and to take all appropriate safety precautions.
To the fullest extent of the law, neither the publisher nor the author assumes
any liability for any injury and/or damage.

The Publisher

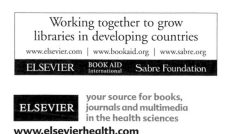

Working together to grow
libraries in developing countries

www.elsevier.com | www.bookaid.org | www.sabre.org

ELSEVIER   BOOK AID International   Sabre Foundation

ELSEVIER   your source for books,
journals and multimedia
in the health sciences
www.elsevierhealth.com

The
publisher's
policy is to use
**paper manufactured
from sustainable forests**

Printed in China

Contents

Preface

Genetics has been the expanding science of the latter half of the 20th century. As we enter the 21st century there are exciting new possibilities for diagnosis and treatment of genetic problems both in man and animals. With our new understanding of genetics married to our knowledge of reproductive physiology it can be said that we are truly beginning to understand the basis of life.

This book is written principally for student veterinary nurses and covers material needed for under-pinning knowledge in genetics and reproductive physiology at level 2 of the Royal College of Veterinary Surgeons' certificate in small animal veterinary nursing. As such it will also be useful for animal technicians and as an introductory text for undergraduate veterinary surgeons.

The material is arranged so that supplementary information or more detailed explanations are provided in text boxes, which can be consulted at once or returned to after the principle point has been grasped. Theory is related to examples and the practical importance of the information is stressed throughout. Each chapter builds upon those preceding but where possible an effort has been made to make each topic stand alone.

Susan Long, 2006

1

The genetic material

Core information: **The genetic material is deoxyribonucleic acid (DNA). The DNA is looped and coiled to form the chromosome. The cell has to first synthesise new DNA before it divides and so there is a cycle of events in the life of a cell – the cell cycle. Most cells divide by a process called mitosis. The gametes are produced by a special cell division called meiosis.**

Living things have characteristics that are either inherited or acquired. Differentiating between the two and understanding how characteristics are inherited is the science of genetics.

Sometimes it is not easy to decide whether a character has been inherited or acquired. For example, in the past, sons tended to follow in their fathers' footsteps – the blacksmith's son was a blacksmith and both had strong muscles. It used to be thought that the son had inherited the strong muscles from his father whereas both had acquired strong muscles because of their way of life, i.e. their environment.

Inherited and acquired characteristics can look the same. The same trait can be inherited in one animal but acquired in another. In general, an inherited characteristic is more common in related animals than unrelated animals. This is true even when related animals are kept under different conditions. Acquired characteristics appear in unrelated animals that are kept in the same manner or are subjected to the same influences. However, acquired characteristics will not be passed on from generation to generation. For example, for safety reasons, farmers often cut the horns off their cows. However, the cows continue to produce calves with horns and they will continue to do so unless the gene for absence of horns (the polling gene) can be introduced into the herd. The presence or absence of horns is an inherited characteristic (Box 1.1).

A characteristic present at birth is said to be a *congenital* characteristic:

■ not all congenital characteristics are inherited
■ not all inherited characteristics are congenital.

Congenital characteristics can be either inherited or acquired, so the mere fact that an animal is born with the trait does not indicate that it is

1

Box 1.1 Polling gene

The gene that causes hornlessness in cattle is called the polling gene. The poll is the part of the head between the ears where the horns are located. The polling gene is represented as P and is dominant to the gene that causes horns to be formed. The horn gene is represented as p. Some breeds, e.g. Aberdeen Angus, that are naturally hornless, are homozygous for the polling gene (PP). The polling gene can be introduced to breeds that naturally have horns, such as the Holstein Friesian, by cross breeding.

Box 1.2 Helix

A helix is a spiral. A double helix is two spirals. For example, if you took an ordinary stepladder and twisted it around a central pole this would produce a double helix and it would very much resemble the structure of DNA.

---

genetic in origin. The characteristic may have been caused by the influence of a chemical during embryonic development.

Not all inherited characteristics are present at birth. Some do not develop until the animal is mature. This is commonly seen in inherited eye defects in dogs.

HISTORICAL DEVELOPMENT OF OUR UNDERSTANDING OF GENETICS

The science of genetics is usually considered to have begun with the experiments of Gregor Mendel, an Austrian monk living in Czechoslovakia, who first described the principles of heredity in the middle of the nineteenth century. However, the importance of his work was not recognised until 1900, long after his death, when biologists began testing his theories, to see if they applied to all plants and animals – they did.

There was another long hiatus until 1944, when it was demonstrated that the genetic information was stored in deoxyribonucleic acid (DNA). It was not until 1953 that Watson and Crick described the double-helix structure of the DNA molecule (Box 1.2). The latter half of the twentieth century saw an explosion of studies into the structure of DNA so that today, whole genomes have been sequenced and numerous genes have been mapped in man and other species.

The study of genetics is now broadly divided into Mendelian genetics, population genetics, molecular genetics and cytogenetics:

- Mendelian genetics deals with inheritance in individuals of characteristics governed by a single gene or just a few genes.
- Population genetics deals with the inheritance of characteristics governed by very many genes. Each gene obeys the principles of Mendelian genetics but because there are so many interacting genes the effect of each individual gene is difficult to predict. Such characteristics are best studied within a group or population of animals, hence the name.
- Molecular genetics is the study of DNA and gene activity at the molecular level.
- Cytogenetics is the study of chromosomes.

STRUCTURE OF DEOXYRIBONUCLEIC ACID (DNA)

It is useful to understand the structure of DNA because this helps in the understanding of genes and their actions.

Structurally, a DNA molecule consists of two parallel chains of atoms joined by cross-links like a stepladder. The chains are the same on both sides and consist of a sugar molecule (deoxyribose) and a phosphate group. The cross-links are formed by two of four bases: adenine (A), thymine (T), guanine (G) and cytosine (C). Adenine always pairs with thymine and guanine always pairs with cytosine. Thus the sequence of bases on one side of the strand determines the sequence of bases on the opposite strand. Each strand is therefore said to be complementary (Fig. 1.1). The 'genetic code' lies in the *sequence of bases* that form the DNA molecule:

- DNA is able to replicate and produce new molecules that are exactly the same as the original.

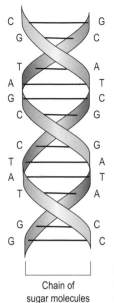

Chain of
sugar molecules

Figure 1.1 Diagram of the structure of deoxyribonucleic acid (DNA). A = adenine, T = thymine, G = guanine, C = cytosine.

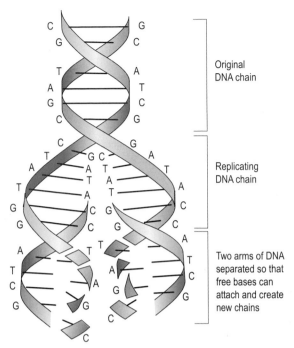

Original DNA chain

Replicating DNA chain

Two arms of DNA separated so that free bases can attach and create new chains

Figure 1.2 Diagram of DNA replication. The chain is 'unzipped' by enzymes and then new bases attach to the 'raw' edges.

Thus it can 'store' the genetic information because of its structure.

■ The size and orientation of the atoms in the DNA molecule means that the structure spirals around its long axis. It therefore forms a double helix.

The molecule can replicate itself exactly by breaking the link between the bases (as if unzipping along the middle of the steps of the ladder) and then adding new units to the broken edges (Fig. 1.2).

Not all DNA codes for something. Much of DNA is non-coding 'rubbish'. The coding sequences of bases are separated by sequences of bases that do not mean anything. The parts of the DNA molecule that code are call *exons* and the non-coding bits in between are called *introns*. In terms of evolution this has the advantage of reducing the chances of any damage to DNA producing damage to a gene.

FORMATION OF CHROMATIN AND CHROMOSOMES

In animals the DNA is found within the nucleus of the cell. In the nucleus the molecules of DNA are coiled around protein; this chain is again coiled to form loops. Coiling enables long lengths of DNA

Box 1.3 DNA coiling

■ DNA loops twice around a histone protein to form a nucleosome (NB the nucleosome is not the gene)
■ The chain of nucleosomes is then concertinaed to form loops
■ The loops are twisted again to form radial loops
■ Finally the radial loops are looped again

to be packed into the relatively small volume of the nucleus. The loops are coiled again to form chromatin (Box 1.3, Fig 1.3). Chromatin is classified as *heterochromatin* and *euchromatin*. The pieces of chromatin are the chromosomes (Box 1.4).

Chromosomes

The chromatin within the nucleus is in a number of separate units, the chromosomes. Each species has a characteristic number of chromosomes, e.g. domestic dogs have a total of 78 chromosomes,

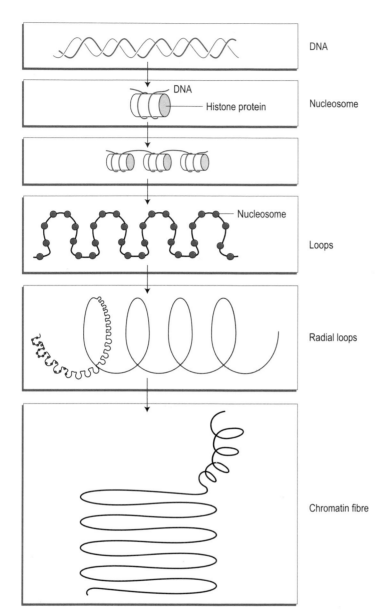

DNA

Nucleosome

Loops

Radial loops

Chromatin fibre

Figure 1.3 Diagram of DNA coiling to form chromatin.

cats have 38 chromosomes and horses have 64 chromosomes. However, this does not mean that different species have different amounts of DNA. In fact, it is approximately the same for all the domestic species, just chopped up into a different number of pieces.

Because individuals receive half their chromosomes from their mother and half from their father, chromosomes are thought of in pairs. Thus dogs have 39 pairs of chromosomes, cats 19 and horses 32 (Box 1.5).

For most of the life of the cell the chromosomes are elongated and are distributed throughout the nucleus, rather like an untidy, tangled ball of pieces of wool. However, when the cell needs to replicate, the chromosomes condense and disentangle and can be seen as separate entities. At one point on the chromosome there is the *centromere*. This looks like a constriction or narrow point and is where the chromosome attaches to the cell spindle when the cell is dividing (Fig. 1.4).

Box 1.4 Heterchromatin and euchromatin

Heterochromatin:
- is darkly staining
- remains tightly coiled (condensed) until the cell divides
- replicates later than euchromatin
- contains very few functional genes

Euchromatin:
- is faintly staining
- contains most of the functional genes

Box 1.5 Chromosome terminology

In an individual, half the chromosomes are inherited from the father (paternal chromosomes) and half from the mother (maternal chromosomes). For this reason chromosomes are usually thought of as in pairs. Each chromosome pair carries similar genes and has the same morphology and is thus said to be *homologous* (*homo* means same).

One pair of chromosomes is known as the sex chromosomes and these do not match each other morphologically; nor do they carry the same genes. All chromosomes that are not the sex chromosomes are known as *autosomes*. Homologous pairs of autosomal chromosomes are morphologically the same and carry the same genes.

THE CELL CYCLE AND CELL DIVISION

The life of a cell can be considered to be cyclical. It does its daily work and then divides. However, before a cell can divide it must synthesise new DNA so that the two new cells have the same amount of DNA as the original (Fig. 1.5):

- The DNA synthesis stage is the S phase. Synthesis seems to be a 'tiring' occupation for a cell because a rest period always follows the S phase.
- This rest phase is called the lag or G_2 phase. After the lag phase the nucleus and cytoplasm divide.
- Division of the nucleus and cytoplasm is the M phase. Once the new cells are formed they can get on with their daily work.

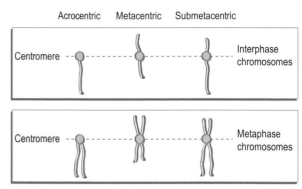

Figure 1.4 Centromeric position on chromosomes. Acrocentric chromosomes have their centromere at one end of the chromosome. Metacentric chromosomes have the centromere in the centre of the chromosome. Submetacentric chromosomes have the centromere towards one end of the chromosome.

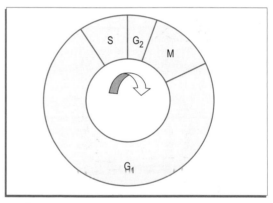

Figure 1.5 The cell cycle. S = synthesis stage. G_2 = lag phase – the interval between DNA synthesis and nuclear division. M = nuclear division (i.e. mitosis or meiosis). G_1 = interphase – the growth phase and interval between the end of nuclear division and the next DNA synthesis.

- The stage when the cell is carrying on its daily work is known as G_1.

For the most part, when a cell divides it produces two new cells that are exact copies of the original. (Thus a better term would be replication or a multiplication division!) This type of cell division is called *mitosis* and occurs when, for example, bones grow or cut skin and blood vessels are repaired. Exact copies of the original cell are produced.

However, the gametes, i.e. the ova and spermatozoa, must have only half the amount of DNA compared to the cells from which they are derived so that when a spermatozoon and an ovum fuse, the new individual has the right amount of DNA again. This type of cell division is called *meiosis* or sometimes, a reduction division. Each new cell has half the amount of DNA as the original cell. It is not a random half, because the new cells have to have one copy of all the chromosomes from the original cell. (The original cell has two copies of each chromosome because one has been inherited from the father and the other from the mother.)

It must be remembered that both types of cell division take place *after* the synthesis stage, i.e. after new DNA has been synthesised. Therefore both types of cell division start with the cell having double the normal amount of DNA. The normal amount of DNA is said to be the *diploid* amount of DNA. Half the normal amount, i.e. that found in the ova and spermatozoa, is the *haploid* amount of DNA.

Mitosis

For convenience of description, mitosis is broken down into a number of stages. However, in practice, each stage flows seamlessly into the next:

- The first stage is *prophase*. At this time the chromosomes begin to condense and become short and fat. The new DNA produced in the S phase and the original DNA are held together at the centromere and so the chromosomes come to look either like an inverted V or like an X. At this stage the chromosomes are still in the nucleus (Fig. 1.6).
- The next stage is called *metaphase*. During this phase the nuclear membrane breaks down and the spindle apparatus forms with a centriole at each pole of the cell. The chromosomes line up in the centre of the cell and the centromere attaches to the fibres of the spindle apparatus. One fibre goes to one pole and the other fibre goes to the other pole (Fig. 1.7).
- The next stage is called *anaphase*. This is when the spindle fibres begin to contract. Since each

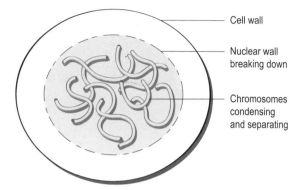

Figure 1.6 Mitotic prophase. The nuclear wall is breaking down and the chromosomes are contracting and separating.

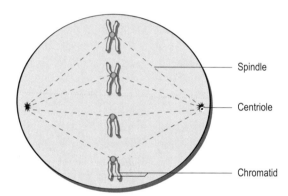

Figure 1.7 Mitotic metaphase. The chromosomes have already synthesised new DNA in the S phase of the cell cycle. The duplicate chromosomes (at this stage called chromatids) are held together at the centromere. They line up on the metaphase plate in the centre of the cell and the spindle fibres attach to the centromere.

centromere has two fibres attached, each pulling in opposite directions, the centromere eventually divides and the two new chromosomes are pulled towards different ends of the cell (Fig. 1.8).
- The final stage is *telophase*. This is when a new nuclear membrane is formed around the cluster of chromosomes to form a nucleus and the spindle fibres disappear. The cytoplasm then divides so that two new cells are formed. The two new cells have the same chromosomes and thus the same genes as the original cell because the DNA had been exactly replicated in the synthesis (S) stage before the nuclear division took place (Fig. 1.9).

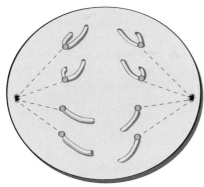

Figure 1.8 Mitotic anaphase. The spindle fibres contract, the centromeres divide and the new chromosomes move to opposite sides of the cell.

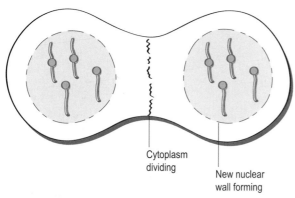

Cytoplasm
dividing

New nuclear
wall forming

Figure 1.9 Mitotic telophase. The cytoplasm begins to divide and new nuclear membranes form around the two new nuclei.

Meiosis

Meiosis is the type of cell division that takes place in the gonads (the ovaries and testes) to produce ova and spermatozoa. It is similar to mitosis, but more complicated because the resulting cells must have half the normal amount of DNA (i.e. the haploid amount). There are in fact two cell divisions in order to halve the number of chromosomes in each final cell.

Once again the process is divided into stages that run into each other. Meiosis has the same stages as mitosis (prophase, metaphase, anaphase and telophase) but the first stage, prophase, is elongated and can take up to four to five days to be completed. It is subdivided into five stages.

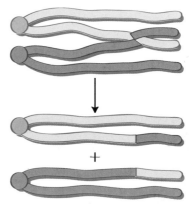

Figure 1.10 Meiotic crossing over. Homologous chromosomes line up next to each other and fuse at certain points, the chiasmata. When the chromosomes part the fused parts have crossed over.

Stages of meiotic prophase 1

- *Leptotene*. During this stage the chromosomes begin to contract.
- *Zygotene*. Chromosomes contract even further. Homologous sets of chromosomes pair up and synaptonemal complexes form. This facilitates crossing over (Box 1.6).
- *Pachytene*. There is further shortening and thickening of the chromosomes. Crossing over takes place at this stage. The crossover point is called the *chiasma*. This is when genetic material from homologous chromosomes is exchanged and is the reason why offspring have genes from maternal and paternal ancestors (Fig. 1.10).
- *Diplotene*. The chromosomes begin to separate and are only held together at the centromere and chiasmata.
- *Diakinesis*. The chromosomes are at their maximum contraction and the chiasmata appear to move towards the end of the chromosomes.

After prophase the next stage is metaphase.

Meiotic metaphase 1

This is similar to mitotic metaphase in that the nuclear membrane breaks down and a spindle forms. The chromosomes line up in the middle of the cell on the metaphase plate. However, after meiotic prophase the homologous chromosomes are still held together at the chiasmata and so in metaphase the homologous chromosomes line up side by side on the metaphase plate instead of underneath one another as in mitotic metaphase. The spindle fibres attach to the centromeres. The spindle fibres from one pole attach to one centromere of one of the pair of homologous chromosomes and the spindle fibres from the other pole attach to the centromere of the other homologous chromosome (Fig. 1.11).

Meiotic anaphase 1

The chiasmata break and the spindle fibres contract. Therefore homologous chromosomes move to opposite poles. Thus anaphase 1 of meiosis differs from mitotic division in that in meiosis this is a separation of homologous chromosomes whilst in mitosis there is a division of centromeres. (Fig.1.12)

Anaphase 1 is followed by a short pause then the cell goes into a mitotic division. Since the chromosomes are already contracted there is no need for another prophase stage and so the cell goes straight into a second metaphase.

Metaphase 2

Since the cytoplasm has not divided there are two groups of chromosomes in the same cell, one on either side. Thus two metaphase plates are formed, along which the centromeres of the chromosomes align. The spindle fibres attach to the centromeres; when they contract the centromeres divide (Fig. 1.13).

Anaphase 2

The contracting spindle fibres cause the centromeres to divide and thus pull the chromatids apart. (Fig.1.14)

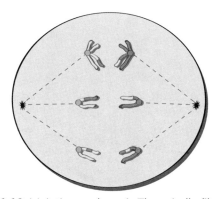

Figure 1.12 Meiotic anaphase 1. The spindle fibres contract and each homologous chromosome moves to opposite sides of the cell.

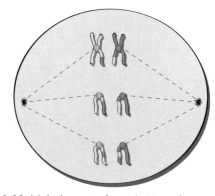

Figure 1.11 Meiotic metaphase 1. Homologous chromosomes line up side-by-side (compared to mitotic metaphase where homologous chromosomes line up below each other) and the spindle attaches to the centromere.

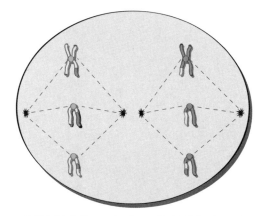

Figure 1.13 Meiotic metaphase 2. At this stage two metaphase plates develop, one on either side of the cell. The chromosomes line up below each other, as in mitotic metaphase, and the two sets of spindle fibres, on either side of the cell, attach to the centromere.

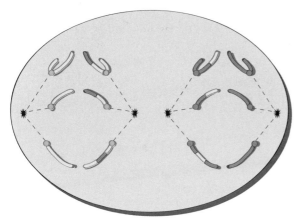

Figure 1.14 Meiotic anaphase 2. The spindle fibres contract and the new chromosomes move apart.

Telophase

After anaphase 2 the cytoplasm divides – this is the telophase stage (Fig. 1.15). The end result of all this activity is that the single cell has replicated its DNA and then divided twice to produce four cells, each of which has half the amount of DNA of the original cell. This is exactly what happens in the testis of the male. One spermatogonium will produce four spermatozoa (Fig. 1.16).

In the female, after anaphase 1, one of the clusters of chromosomes receives very little cytoplasm and fails to divide mitotically. This forms the first polar body. When the second cluster of chromosomes goes through metaphase 2, one of the resulting cells forms the ovum and the other receives very little cytoplasm and forms the second polar body (Fig. 1.17).

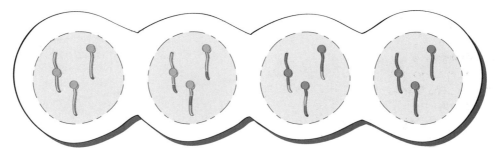

Figure 1.15 Meiotic telophase. A new nuclear membrane develops around each group of chromosomes and the cytoplasm divides between each new nucleus to form four new cells.

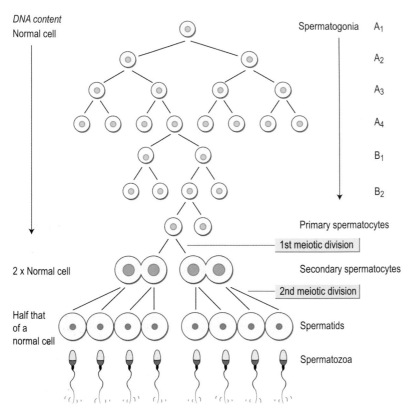

Figure 1.16 Spermatogenesis. Spermatogonia first proliferate and divide mitotically. These are A_1 to A_4 spermatogonia. Thus there is a continuous renewal of spermatogonia. Eventually the spermatogonia begin to divide meiotically. These are called B spermatogonia – they divide mitotically to form primary spermatocytes. The primary spermatocytes undergo the first meiotic division to form secondary spermatocytes. Secondary spermatocytes undergo the second part of meiotic division to form spermatids, which then differentiate into spermatozoa.

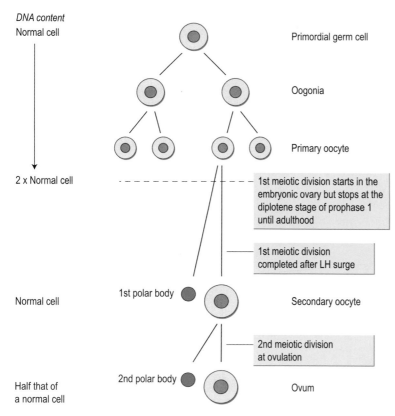

DNA content
Normal cell

Primordial germ cell

Oogonia

Primary oocyte

2 × Normal cell

1st meiotic division starts in the embryonic ovary but stops at the diplotene stage of prophase 1 until adulthood

1st meiotic division completed after LH surge

Normal cell

1st polar body

Secondary oocyte

2nd meiotic division at ovulation

Half that of a normal cell

2nd polar body

Ovum

Figure 1.17 Oogenesis. The primordial germ cell divides mitotically to form oogonia. These divide mitotically again to form primary oocytes. Oocytes start to undergo meiotic division whilst the animal is still an embryo but stop at the diplotene stage. Meiotic division is not completed until just before or just after ovulation, depending upon the species. The first part of the meiotic division of the primary oocyte produces a secondary oocyte plus the first polar body. At fertilisation the meiotic division of the oocyte is completed and the second polar body is formed.

2

Mendelian genetics

Core information: **The genes have defined positions on the chromosomes that are called the gene loci. Genes that are close together on the chromosome are said to be linked. Genes on the sex chromosomes are sex-linked. Alternative forms of genes are said to be alleles and alleles have the same locus. Alleles are formed by mutation. Alleles can interact and be dominant, recessive or co-dominant. Some genes can only be expressed in one sex and these are said to be sex-limited. Non-allelic gene interaction is epistasis. Some gene expression is blocked by other genes, giving rise to incomplete penetrance. Some genes are modified by other genes – this gives rise to variable expressivity.**

Mendelian genetics is concerned with the action of a few genes causing discrete variation. In order to discuss and understand Mendelian genetics a certain amount of new vocabulary has to be learned. The first part of this chapter deals with some of this new terminology. The second part describes the action of some genes as examples of the definitions discussed.

So, what exactly is meant by *discrete variation*?

■ A characteristic shows discrete variation if an animal either has the characteristic (or trait) or it does not (Box 2.1).

Characteristics are coded for by genes. Genes are a specific sequence of bases in the DNA molecule. Each gene sequence is always found in the same position along the DNA. Thus the gene has its own place on a chromosome:

■ The place on the chromosome where the gene is located is called the *gene locus* (Box 2.2).

Chromosomes come in pairs, known as homologous pairs – one from the mother and one from the father. Therefore, there is 'room' for two copies of each gene in the cell, one on each homologous chromosome.

Genes on the same chromosome tend to be inherited together. However, because there is crossing over of homologous chromosome material during meiosis, genes can get separated. The closer together any two genes lie on a chromosome the

---

Box 2.1 Discrete variation

This is when animals either show a characteristic or not. For example, cows either have horns or they do not – there is no gradation to having horns. There can be different types of horns, but the animal either has horns or does not. Thus the characteristic of having horns shows discrete variation.

Box 2.2 Gene locus

Locus means 'exact place'. Thus the gene locus means the place on a specific chromosome where that gene can be found. It is the gene's 'address'. Therefore, every animal of the same species has the same gene at the same locus on the same chromosome.

Different genes have a different locus and no two genes have the same locus. However, alleles of a gene have the same locus because they are alternate forms of the gene and therefore have the same 'address'.

Box 2.3 Gene linkage

In this instance the term *linkage* refers to whether or not different genes at different loci are passed on together. If genes are *linked* it means that they must lie close together on a particular chromosome. It does not mean that they have the same function or even that they interact.

Box 2.4 Sex-linked genes

Genes that are found on the sex chromosomes are said to be sex-linked. Here the term *linkage* tells you about where the gene is located, *not* about the function or action of the gene. Most sex-linked genes have nothing to do with determination of sex, even although they are located on the sex chromosomes. They are normal 'house keeping' genes that allow the cell to function.

In our domestic animals the X chromosome is always much larger than the Y chromosome and so most of the sex-linked genes are on the X chromosome.

---

less likely it is that a crossover event will separate them. Such genes are said to be linked:

- *Gene linkage* is the phenomenon whereby two genes are always inherited together (Box 2.3)
- Those genes that have their loci on the sex chromosomes are said to be *sex-linked genes* (Box 2.4).

Some genes can only be expressed in one sex – the classic example of this is all the genes associated with milk production. The genes are carried by males and females and the male can pass on the genes to male and female offspring – but only the female can express the genes. Such genes are said to be *sex-limited*.

- *Sex-limited* genes are genes whose expression is limited depending on the sex of the animal (Box 2.5).

So far we have discussed genes as if they can only have one structure. However, that is not true.

Box 2.5 Sex-limited genes

Sex-limited genes are on the autosomes. They are not on the sex chromosomes. Here the term *limited* refers to *when* the gene can be expressed. That is, limited to one or other of the sexes.

Sometimes when a cell replicates it does not make an *exact* copy of the old DNA for the new cell. In other words there is a 'mistake' – such a mistake is a *mutation*:

- A *mutation* is when there is a change in the sequence of bases in the DNA molecule.

Mutations are not necessarily bad. Changes in base-pair sequences may have no noticeable effect at all. As we have seen in chapter 1, most of the DNA molecule consists of 'rubbish' sequences and does not consist of functional genes. Thus the chance of a 'mistake' (mutation) occurring where there are genes is reduced and a change in this 'rubbish' DNA will not affect how the cell can code for different characteristics (Box 2.6).

If a mutation does occur in the sequence of bases that form a gene then a number of possible results may occur:

- If the gene is altered to such an extent that it can no longer code for its end product, then the new form of the gene is ineffective in all future cells. If it was a vital gene, one whose loss would mean that the cell could not survive, then a mutation causing such a loss is said to be a *lethal mutation* and the new form of the gene, caused by the mutation, is said to be a *lethal gene*.
- Sometimes the mutation produces a new form of the gene that can still code for the product but the end result is not quite the same as the original. If this mutation has occurred in a spermatogonium or in an oocyte then the changed gene can be passed on to the next generation. In this case the mutation is said to have produced an *allele* of the original gene (Box 2.7).
- All alleles of a gene occupy the same locus on the chromosome as the original gene.

Now, since it is possible to have two copies of a gene in each cell, it means that there can either be two copies of the same allele or one copy of two different alleles. Even if there are many more than two alleles of a gene, it is only possible to have a maximum of two of them in a cell – because there are only two places for the alleles of that gene in a cell. In an individual animal, every cell will have the same two alleles but different animals can have different pairs of alleles. Thus, animals of the same species can differ in many subtle ways.

ALLELIC INTERACTION OR TYPES OF GENE ACTION

Now that we know that there can be different forms of the same gene (i.e. alleles) the next question is, how is the expression of one allele affected by another? Whilst it is easy to see what happens if the two alleles in a cell are the same, what happens if there are two different alleles in a cell? This is

> ### Box 2.6 Mutations affecting the non-coding DNA
>
> It is possible to detect changes in the base-pair sequences and use the existence of such mistakes in non-coding, 'rubbish' DNA as a sort of individual characteristic – a fingerprint. Thus this is a way of identifying an individual – a genetic fingerprint.

> ### Box 2.7 Alleles
>
> An allele is just an alternate form of a gene produced by mutation. Since there can be any number of mutations to the same gene occurring at different times, it follows that there can be any number of alleles for a gene. If there are lots of alleles this is said to be an *allelic series*.
>
> Some genes have no alleles. Other genes have many alleles. It is a chance phenomenon as to how often and where the mutations occur along the DNA molecule.

where the idea of some alleles being dominant and recessive to each other arises.

Alleles may influence the expression, or coding, of each other. Some alleles in a series may block the expression of other alleles in the same series – these are said to be *dominant* alleles and will block the expression of the *recessive* alleles. Thus, recessive alleles have to be present on both homologous chromosomes before they can be expressed. Dominant alleles need only be present on one chromosome because they can block the expression of the recessive alleles on the other chromosome:

- a *dominant* allele will be expressed even if only one copy is present in the genome
- a *recessive* allele is only expressed if two copies are present in the genome.

Not all alleles are either dominant or recessive. Some alleles do not affect the expression of other alleles. In this case when two different alleles are present, both can be expressed. The alleles are therefore said to be *co-dominant*:

■ when two alleles are *co-dominant* both are expressed in the cell.

When there are two different alleles present the cell, or individual, is said to be *heterozygous* for that allele. If the two alleles are the same, then the cell or individual is *homozygous* for the allele (Box 2.8).

INTERACTION OF GENES ON DIFFERENT LOCI

In general a gene and its alleles only influence the expression of alleles on the same locus. However, some genes and their alleles will influence other genes and alleles on a different locus. When genes on different loci interact and affect each other this is said to be *epistasis*.

Epistasis is one of the causes of a phenomenon know as *gene penetrance*. Incomplete gene penetrance occurs when, in a group of animals known to be carrying a gene, some individuals do not exhibit the trait (Box 2.9). Those animals showing the trait do so completely and the trait is entirely absent in other animals. This is different from the situation when there is *variable expressivity*:

■ *variable expressivity* occurs when all animals carrying a gene express the trait but to variable degrees (Box 2.10).

So far we have described genes as having a single effect, i.e. coding for a single product. However, some genes appear to have more than one effect:

■ when a gene appears to affect more than one trait this is *pleiotropism*.
  Pleiotropism may occur because:
■ the gene product is expressed at a number of different points
■ in reality more than one gene is acting but the genes are closely linked and thus are inherited together.

GENE NOMENCLATURE

There are three systems of nomenclature for genes and their alleles but the most commonly used one

---

Box 2.8 Hetero and homo

'Hetero' means different and 'homo' means the same.

Box 2.9 Gene penetrance

The concept of incomplete gene *penetrance* refers to a group of animals, all of which are known to carry a particular gene but only some of which exhibit the trait or characteristic. Thus the gene appears to 'penetrate' and be expressed in some animals but not others. The reasons why some animals carry a gene but do not express it are:

■ Interaction of genes on another locus. That is, animals not expressing the gene in question have another gene on another locus that is blocking the effect of the first gene. This is an epistatic effect.
■ Genotype/environment interactions. In this instance the definition of 'environment' is very wide. It may be the surrounding cells or organ within the animal or the environment surrounding the animal. The environment blocks the expression of the gene and so it cannot 'penetrate.'

Box 2.10 Variable expressivity

The concepts of gene penetrance and variable expressivity are often confused. Gene penetrance is an all-or-nothing effect. The characteristic is either expressed or it is not. With expressivity all animals express the gene but to variable extents. Variable expressivity can be caused by:

■ the characteristic being governed by a number of genes, i.e. the characteristic is *polygenic*
■ genotype/environment interaction

---

in domestic animals is that which denotes a dominant allele by an upper case letter and the recessive allele by a lower case letter, e.g. *B* for black coat colour and *b* for brown coat colour. The *B* allele is dominant to the *b* allele. Thus a black dog would be *BB* if it were homozygous for the black gene or *Bb* if it were heterozygous for the black gene. This is the gene nomenclature used in this book (Box 2.11).

EXAMPLES OF THE PRINCIPLES OF MENDELIAN GENETICS

The first part of this chapter has presented and defined very many new terms relating to Mendelian genetics. The following are some practical examples to help in the understanding of these terms and the basic principles of genetics.

Dominant and recessive genes

Black, chestnut, bay and grey horses
■ Coat colour is due to melanin pigment in the hair and skin.
■ There are two forms of melanin, *eumelanin* and *pheomelanin*. Genes produce coat colour variation by controlling the switch between eumelanin and pheomelanin production.

Box 2.11 Gene nomenclature

Other systems for gene nomenclature are as follows:

■ The system used commonly in mouse genetics is to use a + sign to denote the usual or wild type of gene and then a letter to denote the mutation. The upper case is used if the mutation is dominant to the wild type and a lower case is used if the mutation is recessive to the wild type. For example, if most dogs were black but a few carried a gene for brown then the heterozygous black dog would be denoted +/*b*.
■ Another system uses a capital letter for the gene and then a superscript for the alleles. For example, there are different forms of haemogloblin coded for by different alleles. This can be written Hb^A or Hb^a etc. where Hb is the symbol for haemoglobin, *A* and *a* are the symbols for the alleles and *A* is dominant to *a*.

■ Two alleles govern the proportion of each pigment. The *E* allele (called the extension allele) extends the amount of eumelanin and reduces the proportion of pheomelanin. The result is to produce a black coat in the horse. The other allele is *e* and diminishes the amount of eumelanin and increases the amount of pheomelanin. The result is to produce a brown or chestnut colour – *E* is dominant to *e*.
■ A second gene, *A* (called the agouti gene) shifts any eumelanin to hair of the mane, tail, ear rims and lower leg. The recessive *a* gene allows even expression of eumelanin over the whole body.
■ Thus the *A* and *a* alleles affect the expression of the *E* and *e* gene and are thus showing *epistatic* effects.

So, using the above information, here are a few questions.

(a) What is the genetic make-up of black horses? (Clue: They must have lots of eumelanin and it must be evenly distributed over the whole body.)
(b) What is the genetic make-up of chestnut horses? (Clue: They need pheomelanin and no eumelanin.)
(c) What is the genetic make-up of bay horses? (Clue: Bays have chestnut or brown bodies and black ears, tails and manes.) (Box 2.12).

Polydactyly in cats
Polydactyly is extra toes. Cats usually have four toes on the hind foot and five on the front. Polydactyly in cats is controlled by an autosomal dominant gene (*Pd*) with variable expression. Thus although there is one main gene affecting the condition (*Pd*) there must be other genes that modify the expression. Affected cats have one or two extra toes on the front paws. Exceptionally, cats may have a complete extra set of toes. Polydactyly is more common in cats in the south west of England.

Progressive axonopathy in dogs.
In this condition there are pathological changes in the central nervous system with degeneration of motor nerve fibres. This leads to unco-ordination in the gait and muscular weakness, which becomes

---

Box 2.12 Coat colour genetics in the horse

- Black horses must have lots of eumelanin and therefore must have at least one copy of the *E* allele. To be black all over they must have an even distribution of eumelanin and so must be homozygous for the recessive *aa* alleles. Thus black horses are either *EEaa* or *Eeaa*.
- Chestnut horses need pheomelanin and so must be homozygous for the recessive *e* allele. Since there is no eumelanin it does not matter what agouti alleles the animal has. The agouti alleles do not affect the expression of the pheomelanin. Thus chestnut horses can be *eeAA* or *eeAa* or *eeaa*. Since all chestnut horses are homozygous for the recessive *e* allele, a chestnut mated to a chestnut will always produce a chestnut.
- Bay horses need eumelanin to produce black hair and so need at least one *E* allele; also, the black needs to be on the ears, mane and tail only, so they must have at least one *A* allele. Thus bays are *EEAA* or *EeAA* or *EEAa* or *EeAa*.

Box 2.13 Horse coat colour genetics – action of the *G* allele

The *G* allele causes an accelerated loss of pigment but the pigment is present at birth. Therefore, the foal from a grey horse can be any colour at birth, depending upon which other coat colour genes are present. However, if a foal is carrying the *G* allele, within the first six months of life grey hairs become apparent and the animal can be classified as grey. Complete loss of pigment may take up to two years.

---

evident by about 6 months of age. It is caused by an autosomal recessive gene (*pa*) and seems to be confined to the Boxer breed.

Epistasis

Grey horses

Now that we have mastered two genes in horses which are involved with coat colour, we can consider a third gene, *G*, which causes the accelerated loss of pigment in the hair, irrespective of whether the pigment is eumelanin or pheomelanin. The normal allele, *g*, is recessive to *G* and allows the pigment to remain for the normal period of time. Thus the *G* allele is *epistatic* to both the *E/e* alleles and the *A/a* alleles. All grey horses must have at least one *G* allele. All normal coloured horses must be homozygous for the recessive, non-grey allele, *gg*. Therefore, a non-grey horse mated to a non-grey horse cannot produce a grey foal.

A grey horse does not necessarily have to produce a grey foal because a grey horse can be heterozygous (*Gg*) (Box 2.13).

Variable expression and lethal genes

Manx gene in cats

The Manx breed of cats is well known because they are tail-less. The absence of a tail is due to a mutation *M*, which is dominant to the normal allele *m*. All cats with a tail are homozygous (*mm*) for the normal allele – when two cats with a tail are mated all the kittens will have tails.

The mutant gene *M* causes abnormal development of the skeletal system in general and of the tail and pelvis bones in particular (coccygeal and sacral bones). All Manx cats are heterozygous for the Manx gene and are *Mm*. Homozygous, *MM*, individuals die very early in gestation and so there are no live born *MM* individuals. Thus the Manx allele *M* is said to be a *lethal gene*.

There are in fact four types of Manx cats, classified on the basis of the degree of tail-lessness:

- The true Manx cat is known as a '*rumpy*' and there are no coccygeal vertebrae.
- Some Manx cats have a very few fused tail vertebrae which stand upright from the end of the back. This type is called a '*rumpy-riser*'.
- The third type of Manx cat does have a definite small, tail-like structure made from deformed bones. The 'tail' is very short, kinked and knobbly. This type of Manx cat is called a '*stumpy*'.
- The last form of Manx cats is much more rare. These animals do in fact have a short tail despite being genetically *Mm*. They are called '*longie*'.

It is very obvious, therefore, that the Manx condition has *variable expression*. The variable expression is due to the action of modifying genes that influence the expression of the *manx* gene (Box 2.14).

Folded ears

Normal cats have ears that prick upright. In folded-ear cats the ear is normal at birth but by three months they have become folded down and inward pointing. The condition is inherited as incomplete dominant (*Fd*) and affected animals are hetero-zygotes (*Fdfd*). In the homozygous state there are other abnormalities such as malformed feet and the animals have great difficulty in walking.

Pleiotropism

Cats that are all white are often deaf. The white coat colour is produced by an autosomal dominant gene (*W*) – this gene also affects iris colour and deafness. Not all white cats are deaf and the exact aetiology of the problem is not fully understood.

Mating individuals with different genotypes (Box 2.15)

We have seen that an individual can have different alleles of a gene in its make-up (i.e. be heterozygous at that gene locus) or have the same allele (i.e. be homozygous at that gene locus). That is true for all the gene loci. What we need to consider now is what happens when two individuals are crossed.

The fundamental principles of what happens when two animals are crossed were established by Mendel and are known as Mendel's 1st and 2nd Laws.

- **Mendel's 1st Law** states that alleles separate to different gametes. This means that if an individual is, for example, *Ee* above, then the *E* allele will go to one gamete and the *e* allele will go to the other. You cannot have a normal sperm or egg that has both *E* and *e* (Box 2.16).
- **Mendel's 2nd Law** states that genes on non-homologous chromosomes undergo independent assortment (Box 2.17).

Box 2.15 The genotype and phenotype

The *genotype* of an individual is the genes that the individual has. By contrast the *phenotype* is what the individual looks like. If all the genes were to be expressed then the phenotype would accurately reflect the genotype. However, because of dominance and recession and epistatic and sex-limited effects it is not always possible to guess the genotype from the phenotype.

Box 2.16 Mendel's 1st Law – Alleles separate to different gametes

We now know how this is achieved. It is because the two alleles in an individual are on two different homologous chromosomes, one having been inherited from the mother and the other from the father. During meiosis these chromosomes separate and thus the alleles they carry end up in different gametes. See chapter 1.

Box 2.17 Mendel's 2nd Law – Independent assortment of genes

We can explain Mendel's 2nd law in a similar manner to his first. We know that during meiosis there is crossing over between homologous chromosomes, so some alleles are swapped from one chromatin to another.

Box 2.14 Manx gene in cats

The Manx gene affects all bones in the vertebral column. Anteriorly there is just some shortening of bones but in the more posterior part there can be fusion of, or reduction in, the number of bones. In particular, the sacral and pelvic bones are deformed – as a result Manx cats have an abnormal gait. In some instances the pelvic deformity results in narrowing of the digestive tract leading to partial or complete blockage. The deformed vertebral column can also lead to damage to the spinal nerves. Therefore the Manx gene is not only lethal in the homozygous state but also semi-lethal in the heterozygous state.

We can work out the result of crossing any two individuals by means of a Punnet square. This is simply a square down one side of which is listed the possible gametes of the male and on the top of which is listed the possible gametes of the female. For example, let us consider just three genes

■ gene A with two alleles *A* and *a*
■ gene B with two alleles *B* and *b*
■ gene D with two alleles *D* and *d*.

If we cross a male whose genetic make-up is *Aa,bb,Dd* with a female who is *aa,Bb,Dd* what genetic make-up would the offspring have? To answer this we have to first work out all the possible combinations of genes in the sperm from the male and the genes in the egg of the female – then we can see what would result when the sperm fertilises the egg. So, from Mendel's first law we know that we must have one allele of each of the genes in each gamete.

Therefore, for the suggested mating above:

■ the [*Aa,bb,Dd*] male will produce sperm with

(*abD*) or (*abd*) or (*AbD*) or (*Abd*)

■ The [*aa,Bb,Dd*] female will produce eggs with

(*aBD*) or (*aBd*) or (*abD*) or (*abd*).

In this example the male and female each have four different possible genotypes for the gametes. We can now work out the genetic make-up of the offspring using a Punnet square (Fig. 2.1).

This particular mating produces 12 different possible combinations of genotypes for the offspring. If the original male and female were heterozygous for alleles of all three genes then the possible number of genotypes of the offspring would be 27! Fortunately, you do not have to remember this because there is a neat formula:

If the number of gene pairs is *n*, then the possible number of gametes is 2^n and the number of possible genotypes in the offspring is 3^n.

Thus, with two gene pairs, *Aa,Bb*, *n* = 2 and so the number of gametes is 4 (2^2) and the number of offspring genotypes is 9 (3^2). With three gene pairs, *Aa,Bb,Dd*, *n* = 3 and thus the number of gametes is 8 (2^3) and the number of offspring genotypes is 27 (3^3). Try drawing a Punnet square and working it out!

	Female gametes:	aBD	aBd	abD	abd
	abD	aaBbDD	aaBbDd	aabbDD	aabbDd
Male gametes:	abd	aaBbDd	aaBbdd	aabbDd	aabbdd
	AbD	AaBbDD	AaBbDd	AabbDD	AabbDd
	Abd	AaBbDd	AaBbdd	AabbDd	Aabbdd

Figure 2.1 Example of a punnet square.

3

Simple Mendelian patterns of inheritance

Chapter contents

Core information: **Genes and alleles with different interactions show a particular pattern of inheritance. It is therefore possible to examine a pedigree and from the pattern of expression of a characteristic in the different generations deduce whether the characteristic is inherited and what form of gene action is occurring.**

IS IT INHERITED?

When a characteristic or trait is encountered for the first time it can be difficult to determine whether the effect is genetic, and therefore heritable, or whether it is due to external factors which are not genetic in origin. When an external or environmental factor produces a phenotype which is identical to that produced by a gene the external factor is said to have produced a *phenocopy*, i.e. a copy of the phenotype (Box 3.1)

If a characteristic is caused by genes, then the incidence of the characteristic will be higher in related individuals than unrelated individuals. This is because related individuals are more likely to have similar genes than unrelated individuals. One way of investigating whether a condition or characteristic is inherited is to look at pedigrees and see when and how often the condition or characteristic appears.

The different types of gene action are autosomal dominant, autosomal recessive, sex-linked dominant and sex-linked recessive. Each of these gene actions produces a pattern of affected individuals within a pedigree. This pattern can be used to try and determine what type of gene is producing a particular effect.

Autosomal dominant genes

Characteristics that are caused by dominant genes will be expressed in every individual carrying the gene. It does not matter whether there is only one copy of the gene or two. Furthermore, any autosomal gene is just as likely to be inherited by a male or female – so the incidence of the characteristic is the same in males as females. Thus the pattern of inheritance for autosomal dominant genes can be listed as follows:

Box 3.1 Phenocopy

A phenocopy is when a characteristic can be produced due to a gene effect or an external environmental effect. An extreme example of this would be a tail-less cat. A cat can be born with no tail because of the Manx gene (*M*) or because of the action of certain chemicals during its gestation, or because the mother cat accidentally bit off the tail at birth. In each case the cat would be tail-less and so they would be *phenocopies* – but only the cat with the Manx gene could possibly pass the characteristic on to its offspring.

- The defect is transmitted from generation to generation without skipping a generation.
- Every affected offspring must have at least one affected parent (except in the case of a new mutation).
- Normal offspring from affected parents will not be carrying the gene and so will produce normal offspring if they are mated to normal individuals. In other words, normal offspring from affected parents cannot pass on the condition.
- Approximately equal numbers of male and female individuals will be affected if an extensive enough pedigree is available.
- If the condition is rare but not lethal then matings producing an affected individual will usually have been a normal individual crossed with a heterozygous-affected individual – i.e. *aa* (normal) × *aA* (heterozygous affected). In this case the ratio of normal to affected offspring will be 1 in 2 or 50:50.

Autosomal recessive genes

Recessive genes will only be expressed in individuals that have two copies, i.e. are homozygous for the gene. Therefore if an individual has only one copy it is possible for the gene to be passed from generation to generation without being revealed until at last an individual receives two copies of the gene and the condition is expressed.

Again, any autosomal gene is just as likely to be inherited by males and females and so the incidence of the condition is the same in males and females. Thus, the pattern of inheritance of autosomal recessive conditions is as follows:

- The disorder may skip a generation.
- *All* offspring of two affected parents will be affected (because all offspring will be homozygous).
- Approximately equal numbers of male and female individuals will be affected if an extensive enough pedigree is available.
- If the disorder is rare:
  1. Most affected individuals will have two normal parents. i.e. the parents will be heterozygous carriers of the recessive (*Aa*).
  2. Most normal parents producing affected offspring will be more closely related than other animals in the population. This is because normal animals producing an affected offspring must be carriers of the recessive and if the gene is rare then two animals carrying the gene are likely to be related.
  3. If both parents are heterozygous carriers (*Aa* × *Aa*) then the segregation ratio of affected offspring (*aa*) will be 1 in 4.
  4. Matings between an affected and an unrelated normal animal will usually produce only normal offspring. This is because an unrelated normal animal is not likely to be a heterozygous carrier and so such a mating will be *aa* (affected) × *AA* (normal) and produce only normal but carrier animals (*Aa*).

X-linked dominant genes

X-linked genes are genes located on the X chromosome. Dominant genes are genes that will be expressed even if there is only a single copy of the gene, i.e. only one X chromosome is carrying the gene. Thus the pattern of inheritance of X-linked dominant genes is as follows:

- All animals carrying the gene will express the gene. Therefore a normal individual cannot be carrying the gene.
- Every affected offspring must have at least one affected parent.
- Affected males when mated to normal females will not pass the gene to any of their sons. This

is because sons receive their Y chromosome from their father (and their X chromosome from their mother). Therefore none of the sons will receive any X-linked gene from their father.

- Affected males when mated to normal females will pass the gene to all the daughters. This is because daughters always receive their father's X chromosome (and one X chromosome from their mother). Thus all the daughters will receive any X-linked gene from their father.

- If the condition is rare then the incidence of the defect or disease in females is approximately twice that in males. This is because females have two X chromosomes and therefore have twice the chance of having the X-linked gene compared with males.

X-linked recessive genes

X-linked genes are located on the X chromosome. Recessive genes will normally only be expressed if there are two copies of the gene. With X-linked recessive genes in males, which only have one X chromosome, there is no second copy possible. However, this does not matter because there is no second *dominant gene* to mask the recessive, thus the recessive can be expressed. Thus the pattern of inheritance of X-linked recessive genes is as follows:

- The defect or disease may skip a generation. This is because if the gene causing the disorder is passed to a female she may have a normal gene on the other X chromosome.
- All offspring of affected parents will be affected.
- The incidence of the disease or defect is lower in females than males. This is because if females (who always have two X chromosomes) only have one copy of the gene it can be masked by the normal gene on the second X chromosome. However, in the male, if their X chromosome carries the X-linked recessive gene it will always be expressed.
- If the defect is rare then
  1. Most affected individuals will be males.
  2. They will result from normal parents (but the female will be a carrier).

3. Affected *males* when mated to normal females will not transmit the disease *or* disorder but half their daughters will be carriers. This is because sons will not receive their father's X chromosome and so will not have the disease but daughters will have one normal X chromosome from their mother, which will mask the gene causing the disorder on the X chromosome from their father – since they do have the gene from their father they will be carriers (Box 3.2).

4. Affected *females* when mated to normal males will transmit the disease or defect to all their sons. None of their daughters will show the disease or defect but they will all be carriers. They will not show the disease because they will have the normal X chromosome from their normal father and this will mask the X-linked recessive on the X chromosome from the mother (Box 3.3).

Box 3.2 Example of a male with an X-linked recessive gene mating with a normal female

Normal gene = A, recessive allele = a
$X^a Y$ (affected male) × $X^A X^A$ (normal female)
The punnet square for this mating is:

		Male gametes:	X^a	Y
Female gametes:		X^A	$X^A X^a$	$X^A Y$
		X^A	$X^A X^a$	$X^A Y$

$X^A Y$ is a normal male and $X^A X^a$ is a carrier female

Box 3.3 Example of affected female mated to a normal male

Normal gene = A, recessive allele = a
$X^A Y$ (normal male) × $X^a X^a$ (affected female)
The punnet square for this mating is:

		Male gametes:	X^A	Y
Female gametes:	X^a		$X^a X^A$	$X^a Y$
	X^a		$X^a X^A$	$X^a Y$

$X^a Y$ are affected males and $X^a X^A$ are carrier females

DETERMINATION OF WHETHER AN ANIMAL IS A CARRIER OF A RECESSIVE GENE

Pedigree analysis will be able to tell you which animals are carrying a dominant gene and which animals are homozygous for a recessive gene. However, it is not always possible to tell from the pedigree whether an animal is a carrier of a recessive gene. Neither is it possible to tell whether an animal is a carrier of a recessive gene just by its phenotype.

In order to determine whether an animal is a carrier of a recessive gene test matings have to be carried out. The suspect carrier can be mated to a known homozygous animal. This is called *the backcross to the recessive*. In this case, there is a 50% chance of any offspring being homozygous for the recessive gene if the test animal is a carrier. If the test animal is not a carrier then no offspring will be homozygous for the recessive gene. The big question is how many normal offspring need to be born before you can be sure that the test animal is not going to produce a homozygous recessive offspring? The strict answer is that it would have to be an infinite number! This is obviously not useful. However, we can use the principles of probability and say that if there are *seven normal* offspring, then we can be 99% sure that the test animal is not a carrier of the recessive (Box 3.4).

Now, it is not always going to be possible to carry out a test mating with a known homozygous animal. For example, homozygous animals may not be able to breed. In these circumstances the test mating has to be done with a known carrier. A known carrier would be one that has already produced a homozygous recessive animal. This time, if you carry out a backcross to a known carrier (heterozygous animal) then, on the basis of probability, you need to have *16 normal* offspring before you can be 99% sure that the test animal is not a carrier (Box 3.5).

Box 3.4 Backcross to a known homozygous recessive

Let us assume that the test animal is a carrier of a recessive gene *a*. Then the test mating will be:
Aa (test animal) × *aa* (known homozygous recessive animal)
The punnet square for this mating is:

Test animal's gametes:		*A*	*a*
Recessive animal's gametes:	*a*	*Aa*	*aa*
	a	*Aa*	*aa*

Thus the chance of any offspring of such a mating being normal is 50% or $^1/_2$. The chance that two successive offspring will be normal is $^1/_2 \times ^1/_2$. The chance that three successive offspring will be normal is $^1/_2 \times ^1/_2 \times ^1/_2$ and so on. Thus, if you have seven normal offspring, the chances of this happening and the test animal being a carrier is:

$$^1/_2 \times ^1/_2 \times ^1/_2 \times ^1/_2 \times ^1/_2 \times ^1/_2 \times ^1/_2$$

which is 0.0078. This is 0.01 correct to two decimal places. Put another way, this will only happen by chance once in a hundred times. Therefore we can be 99% sure that if there are seven normal offspring with such a mating, the test animal is not carrying the recessive gene. Of course, the birth of only one offspring that is homozygous shows that the test animal was a carrier of the recessive gene.

Box 3.5 Backcross to a known heterozygous carrier of a recessive

Let us assume that the test animal is a carrier of a recessive gene *a*. Then the test mating will be:
Aa (test animal) × *Aa* (known heterozygous carrier of the recessive)
The punnet square for this mating is:

Gametes of the test animal:		*A*	*a*
Gametes of the known carrier of the recessive:	*A*	*AA*	*Aa*
	a	*Aa*	*aa*

Thus the chance of any offspring from this mating appearing normal is 75% or $^3/_4$. The chance that two successive offspring will be normal is $^3/_4 \times ^3/_4$. The chance of three successive normal offspring is $^3/_4 \times ^3/_4 \times ^3/_4$ and so on. The chance of 16 successive offspring being normal is 0.01 – there is only one chance in a hundred that this will happen if the test animal is a heterozygous carrier of the recessive.

4

Cytogenetics

> *Core information:* **Chromosomes can be seen with an ordinary light microscope. Individual chromosomes are best examined during mitotic metaphase. Meiotic chromosomes are more easily viewed in males than females because most of the meiotic stages in the female take place when the individual is a fetus. The types of chromosomal abnormalities can be divided into numerical, structural and mixed cell lines.**

Cytogenetics is the study of chromosomes. Chromosomes can be seen under a normal light microscope. Therefore, with appropriate preparation and staining it is possible to examine their number and morphology. In a normal, non-dividing cell the chromosomes are elongated and entwined round one another and therefore it is very difficult to identify individual chromosomes. However, in certain circumstances it is possible to identify an X chromosome in non-dividing cells.

THE SEX CHROMATIN OR BARR BODY

In some interphase cells it is sometimes possible to recognise one of the X chromosomes in a female. This is because whilst one X chromosome is elongated like the autosomes, the other X chromosome of the female remains contracted even in the interphase cell. It forms a dot-like feature in the nucleus called the *Barr body* (named after one of the people who first noticed it). It is also called the *sex chromatin* because it is now known that the dot is chromatin formed by one of the X chromosomes. It is not seen in the male because the normal male only has one X chromosome and this remains elongated. In animals with more than one X chromosome the other X chromosomes are always contracted and form Barr bodies. The sex chromatin/Barr body is most easily seen in cells from the dorsal root ganglion of the spinal cord. However, this is not a very convenient place to look! In humans, and to a lesser extent cats and dogs, it is also possible to see the sex chromatin/Barr body in cells from the lining of the mouth. To look for the sex chromatin/Barr body one can take a buccal smear and stain the cells. (This was one of the first ways we had to check the genetic sex of human athletes in the 1950s and early 1960s.)

DRUMSTICK APPENDAGE

In animals such as cattle and sheep, which have keratinised cells lining the mouth, it is not really possible to identify the sex chromatin/Barr body from buccal smears. A more convenient source of cells is white blood cells. The sex chromatin is not visible in most cells but in the nucleus of some polymorphonucleocytes the contracted X chromosome forms a mass that looks like a chicken leg or *drumstick appendage* as it is known (Fig. 4.1). However, just being able to tell how many X chromosomes there are is very limited cytogenetic information.

METAPHASE CHROMOSOMES

To examine the whole chromosome complement in a cell it is best to examine chromosomes during mitotic metaphase. Thus techniques have been developed to induce cells to divide and then to stop them at mitotic metaphase. The most easily

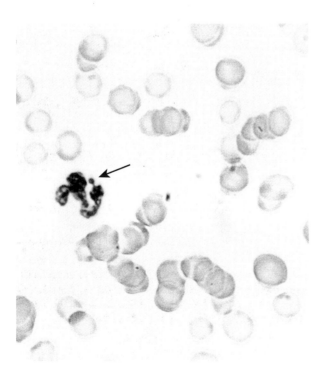

Figure 4.1 A blood smear from a cat showing a polymorphonucleocyte with a drumstick appendage (arrowed).

sourced cells are peripheral blood lymphocytes and so most chromosomes are examined by taking a blood sample, culturing the cells for two or three days, stopping the cells at mitotic metaphase and then fixing them. When this cell suspension is dropped onto a microscope slide the cell wall breaks and the chromosomes are spread out on the slide (Fig. 4.2). The photograph can be cut up and the chromosomes arranged in an internationally agreed order to produce a karyotype (Fig. 4.3). The metaphase can be stained in various ways so that individual chromosomes and even particular parts of chromosomes can be identified (Fig. 4.4).

MEIOTIC CHROMOSOMES

It is possible to see individual chromosomes during meiotic division but there is really only a ready source of cells in the post-pubescent male (Fig. 4.5). Most of the stages of meiosis in the female take place in the embryo and are completed only shortly before or just after ovulation of the egg.

Once reliable techniques were developed to visualise chromosomes it became possible to differentially stain them and characterise small segments of each chromosome. The commonest differential stain is *G banding* which produces a barcode-like effect along the length of the chromosome – unique for each homologous pair of

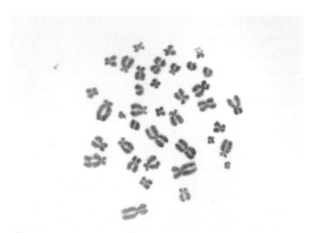

Figure 4.2 Metaphase spread from a cat. A cat has a total of 38 chromosomes.

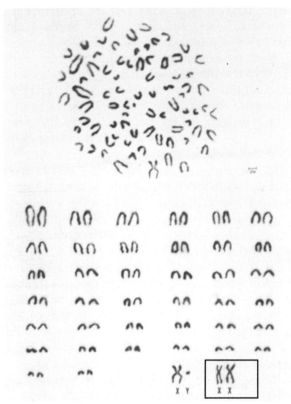

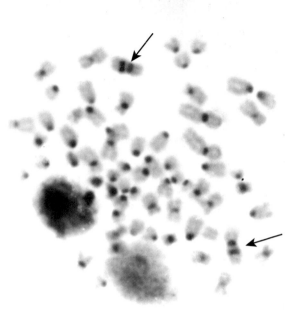

Figure 4.4 Metaphase chromosomes from a horse. The chromosomes have been 'C-banded', which is one of the differential stains to show heterochromatin. The X chromosome (arrowed) has an interstitial c-band in the long arm and so can easily be identified.

Figure 4.3 Metaphase spread and karyotype of a dog. The dog has a total of 78 chromosomes in each cell. This chromosome spread is from a male. A female would have XX sex chromosomes (boxed) instead of the X and Y chromosomes.

chromosomes. The latest molecular genetic technique for staining chromosomes links a dye or stain to a specific piece of DNA to produce a *chromosome paint*. Such techniques allow the identification of normal chromosomes and any deviation from the normal. Chromosomal abnormalities have been associated with gross deformities and/or infertility in animals due to damage or loss of genes in the abnormal chromosome.

CHROMOSOMAL ABNORMALITIES

Chromosomal abnormalities can be divided into numerical abnormalities, structural abnormalities and multiple cell lines. Again it is necessary to learn some new terminology to understand some of the abnormalities.

HORSE

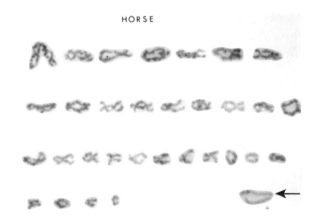

Figure 4.5 Karyotype of a cell from a horse in meiotic prophase at the diplotene/diakinesis stage. Homologous chromosomes can be seen paired and entwined. The sex chromosomes (arrowed) do not entwine.

Box 4.1

Diploid implies two (because 'di' usually means two) but the term is used because the chromosomes come in pairs, one from the father and one from the mother. These are known as homologous pairs.

Numerical abnormalities

- The normal number of chromosomes in a cell is called the *diploid* number (Box 4.1).
- Any deviation from the diploid number is known as *heteroploidy*.
- Ova and spermatozoa (i.e. the germ cells) only have one of each of the homologous pairs of chromosomes and therefore their normal number of chromosomes is half the diploid number, which is called the *haploid* number of chromosomes.
- Cells which have whole multiples of the haploid number of chromosomes above the diploid are called *polyploid* cells, e.g. three times the haploid is *triploidy*, four times is *tetraploidy* etc.
- Cells which have a few chromosomes more or less than the diploid number for the species are *aneuploid* cells. In general it is easier for a cell to cope with too much genetic material than too little.
- Where one of a homologous pair of chromosomes is missing this is called *monosomy*.
- A cell with an extra chromosome of a homologous pair is said to be *trisomic* for that chromosome.

Structural abnormalities

Breakage of genetic material occurs quite frequently. The normal repair mechanisms quickly rectify the damage and the repaired chromosome is unchanged. However, sometimes, the repair cannot take place or is incorrect.

The simplest of all structural abnormalities is a *deletion*, i.e. there is a break in the chromosome that fails to repair and some genetic material is lost. If the lost material contains a gene essential to life then the deletion is lethal. If it is not lethal it may inhibit normal development so that an abnormality in the animal is seen. In some cases, if the lost genetic material does not contain a coding gene (i.e. it is heterochromatin) then the loss of genetic material may have no effect at all.

The next type of abnormality is a *translocation*. That is, the genetic material is not lost but moved to a new place. The new place can be within the original chromosome or on another chromosome. Translocations arise because there has been a breakage within one or more chromosomes and there is a mis-repair. There are a number of different types of translocations. In general, a translocation does not affect the function of the animal that is carrying the translocation because no genetic material is lost. However, when the animal tries to make gametes (sperm or ova) pairing up during meiosis Is compromised and the result is that the fertility of the individual is reduced. The degree of reduction in fertility depends on the type of translocation and the particular genetic material involved in the rearrangement (Fig. 4.6).

Multiple cell lines

A chromosome abnormality can occur in a single cell, in a number of cells or in all the cells in the body. If the animal has some normal cells and cells with a chromosomal abnormality then the animal is said to be *mixoploid* i.e. it has a mixture of cells. If this mixture of cells comes from one original cell line then the animal is said to be a *mosaic*. If the mixture of cells derives from two cell lines then the animal is said to be a *chimera*. A chromosomal abnormality will only be passed on to an animal's offspring if it occurs in the sperm or ova.

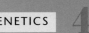

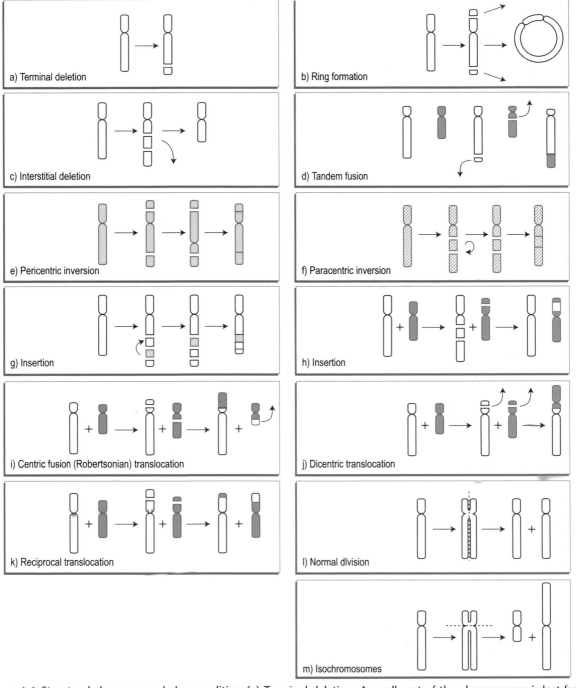

Figure 4.6 Structural chromosomal abnormalities. (a) Terminal deletion. A small part of the chromosome is lost from one end. (b) Ring formation. If there is a terminal deletion from both ends of a bi-armed chromosome then the 'raw' ends may join to form a ring. (c) Interstitial deletion. When there are two breaks in a chromosome the middle piece may be lost before there is a repair. (d) Tandem fusion. If a break occurs in one chromosome near the centromere and then the centromere is lost the free part of the chromosome may attach to a broken end of a second chromosome. (e) Pericentric inversion. Here there is a break either side of the centromere in a bi-armed chromosome and the middle piece inverts before the chromosome is repaired. (f) Paracentric inversion.

Figure 4.6 caption overleaf Here there are two breaks near the centromere and the central piece rotates through 180° before the repair is achieved. (g) Insertion. If there are three breaks, there may be a rearrangement within the chromosome without any loss of genetic material. (h) Insertion. If there are two breaks in one chromosome and one break in another the free piece in the first chromosome may be inserted into the broken ends of the second chromosome. (i) Centric fusion translocation. This was once named a Robertsonian translocation after the person who first described the rearrangement. In this rearrangement there is a loss of a small amount of genetic material. In one chromosome the loss involves the centromere and in the other chromosome, a small part near the centromere. The result is a reduction in the total number of chromosomes because two chromosomes have joined together.
(j) Dicentric chromosomes. This is similar to a centric fusion. If there is a break very near the centromere in two chromosomes, the broken ends may fuse and create one large chromosome but with two centromeres.
(k) Reciprocal translocation. In this abnormality there is a break in two non-homologous chromosomes and the free pieces are swapped before the chromosomes are repaired. There is no actual loss of genetic material, it is just re-arranged and will cause problems at meiosis if the damage has occurred in a spermatocyte or oocyte.
(l) Isochromosome. During anaphase the centromere usually divides in the vertical plane. This results in two new identical chromosomes. If the centromere divides in the horizontal plane two abnormal chromosomes are formed.

5

The sex chromosomes and sex differentiation

Core information: **The sex chromosomes are the X and Y chromosomes. Males are XY and females are XX. The Y chromosome carries male-determining genes. They trigger a cascade of genes that convert the undifferentiated embryo into a male. The female is the 'default sex'. She develops in the absence of the male-determining genes.**

SEX CHROMOSOMES

The sex chromosomes are the X and Y chromosomes. The female has an XX sex chromosome complement and the male has an XY sex chromosome complement.

The X chromosome carries a number of genes but most are not involved with sex determination. They are what can be called 'housekeeping' genes, i.e. genes involved with the everyday life of the cell or individual. As well as a large number of genes there is heterochromatin, i.e. chromatin that does not contain coding genes, and so in our domestic species the X chromosome is usually quite a large chromosome.

By contrast, the Y chromosome contains few genes that are not related to sex determination and in most of our domestic animals (e.g. cats, dogs, horses, donkeys, cattle, sheep, goats and pigs) there is very little heterochromatin. Thus the Y chromosome is usually quite a small chromosome (Box 5.1).

GENE DOSAGE COMPENSATION THEORY (THE LYON HYPOTHESIS OF X INACTIVATION)

Since females have two X chromosomes and the X chromosome is larger and carries many more genes than the Y chromosomes, it might be suspected that the male with an XY complement is deficient in the 'dose' of genes it inherits relative to the female. However, there is not a problem because in the female, one of the X chromosomes becomes highly condensed and inactivated. Chromatin thus

---

Box 5.1 Different types of sex chromosomes

Some animals have a more complicated sex chromosome complement than the simple XX/XY system. For example, the hamster has the normal XX for female and XY for the male but both the X and Y chromosomes have large blocks of heterochromatin, which make each chromosome much bigger than in the normal system. This does not matter because heterochromatin does not contain coding genes.

Even more unusual is the gerbil. Here, the X chromosome has translocated to (i.e. become attached to) one of the autosomes. There is a separate Y chromosome as normal so the female is AX + AX (where A stands for the autosome) and the male is AX + Y + A and so has an odd number of chromosomes. This arrangement again is not a problem because no genetic material has been lost, just rearranged!

---

contracted is said to be *facultative heterochromatin*. ('Facultative' because it has the facility to return to active euchromatin.) This is called the 'Lyon hypothesis of X inactivation and gene dosage compensation' named after the person who first put forward the idea.

At fertilisation, and for a short time during early embryonic development, both X chromosomes are functional and their genes are active. Soon, however, one of the X chromosomes ceases to function. The decision as to which X chromosome becomes inactive in the cell is a random process. However, thereafter, when the cell nucleus multiplies and divides to form new cells, the same X chromosome remains inactivated.

Not quite all the X chromosome becomes inactivated. There is a small part that contains 'house keeping' genes and these same genes are also found on the Y chromosome. This part of the X and Y chromosome is called the *pseudoautosomal region* and is the only part of the sex chromosomes that pair up during meiosis. In this way there is very little chance of any of the sex-determining genes on the Y chromosome crossing over to the X chromosome during meiosis.

SEX DIFFERENTIATION

The male

Sex differentiation starts in the early embryo. In mammals, the Y chromosome carries the primary male-determining genes, the main one of which is the 'testis-determining gene' (Tdy) or 'sex-determining region' (SRY). This gene controls the expression of a number of other genes – some also on the Y chromosome but also some on the autosomes. The effect of the expression of the Tdy gene is that the undifferentiated gonad develops as a testis.

- In the XY embryo the undifferentiated gonad support cells direct the gonads to differentiate into a testis (note that it is not the germ cells but their support cells that do this).
- A meiotic inhibition substance is secreted and the germ cells do not undergo meiotic division in the embryo (indeed, there is no meiotic division until puberty).
- Once the testis has differentiated the Sertoli cells produce a Mullerian Inhibition Substance (MIS). This blocks the development of the Mullerian duct system – the female reproductive duct system. Later the Leydig cells secrete testosterone, which stimulates the Wolffian duct system – the male reproductive duct system (Box 5.2).
- At puberty a spermatogenesis gene on the Y chromosome of spermatogonia starts spermatogenesis by stimulating meiotic division.

Thus, the male phenotype requires a *positive* stimulus to develop.

The female

In the female, development happens by *default*. That is, because male development is *not* directed, female development occurs.

- In the XX embryo there is no suppression of meiosis and so germ cells in the undifferentiated gonads begin meiosis and cells orientate themselves into the morphology of an ovary with a medulla and cortex. (The oogonia do not complete the full meiotic process and cells

Mullerian	*Wolffian*
cranial (anterior) vagina	penis
cervix	penile urethra
uterus	seminal vesicles
uterine horns	vas deferens
uterine tubes (Fallopian tubes)	epididymis

Box 5.3 **Coat colour genetics in the cat – patches of white fur**

The white fur is not associated with the genetics of tortoiseshell coat colour but many tortoiseshell cats have a gene that causes patches of white fur to develop. The white areas are controlled by a separate, autosomal 'white gene', the effect of which is to over-ride all other coat colour genes in certain areas of the body, e.g. under the chin and along the ventral abdomen.

remain resting at diplotene until just before ovulation in the post pubertal animal.)

- In the absence of any suppression the Mullerian ducts develop and so the female duct system is established. [The cranial (anterior) vagina is part of the Mullerian duct system but the caudal (posterior) vagina develops by in-budding from the perineal region. The inbudding forms the urogenital sinus, from which develops the caudal (posterior) vagina and vestibule.]

TORTOISESHELL CATS

The tortoiseshell coat colour in cats is a mixture of orange (ginger) and tabby or black. Many tortoiseshell cats also have patches of white fur but this is not an essential characteristic of the tortoiseshell coat colour. In America, cats with the three colours are known as 'tricolors' or Calico cats.

The tortoiseshell coat colour arises because the orange gene is sex-linked and epistatic to the autosomal black or tabby genes. Tortoiseshell female cats are heterozygous for the orange gene, i.e. one X chromosome has the orange gene and one does not. Therefore, their sex chromosome complement can be written $X^o X^-$ where X^o is the X chromosome carrying the orange gene and X^- is the X chromosome without the orange gene.

In the $X^o X^-$ female only one X chromosome is functional in each cell as usual. In the cell where the functional X chromosome is the one carrying the orange gene, this gene will suppress the black or tabby gene and only the orange hair colour will be produced. In cells where the functional X chromosome is the one without the orange gene then the black or tabby gene (whichever one is

present) will be allowed to be expressed. Since inactivation of one of the X chromosomes does not take place until about day 12 of embryogenesis in the cat, there are patches or blocks of skin cells that have the same active X chromosome. This results in patches of orange or patches of tabby or black. Thus the tortoiseshell cat is a good example of sex-linked genes and epistatic effects (Box 5.3).

Male tortoiseshell cats

Since the tortoiseshell coat colour requires the presence of two X chromosomes (one carrying the orange gene, X^o, and one not, X^-) it would seem that it is not possible to have male tortoiseshell cats. Nevertheless, male tortoiseshell cats do occur. When such animals have been examined they have been found to be chromosomally abnormal. They do have two X chromosomes, either in every cell of the body, in which case their sex chromosome complement is XXY, or there are two distinct cell lines, e.g. XX/XY or XX/XXY or XY/XXY etc. There must be at least one cell line with a Y chromosome for the animal to develop as a phenotypic male (Boxes 5.4, 5.5). Most male tortoiseshell cats are infertile. However, those animals with a normal male cell line (i.e. 38,XY) may be fertile (Figs 5.1, 5.2).

ABNORMALITIES OF SEX DIFFERENTIATION

There are a number of different ways for sex differentiation to go wrong:

Box 5.4 Some examples of chromosome complements in male tortoiseshell cats

38,XX/38,XY

Two cell lines, i.e. chimera – one a normal female, the other a normal male. Some cats with this chromosome complement have been fertile.

39,XXY

Single cell line – every cell has one extra X chromosome. This clinical presentation is called the Klinefelter syndrome after the person who first described it.

38,XX/39,XYY

Two cell lines, i.e. chimera – one normal female line and the other where every cell had an extra Y chromosome.

38,XY/57,XYY

Two cell lines – one was a normal male line and the other was trisomic, i.e. there were three copies of each chromosome in each cell.

38,XY/39XXY/40XXYY

Three cell lines – one normal male line, one line where each cell has an extra X chromosome and one line where each cell has two extra X chromosomes.

Box 5.5 Fertility of male tortoiseshell cats

Most male tortoiseshell cats are infertile. Male tortoiseshell cats with the chromosome complement of 39,XXY are infertile because the extra X chromosome in spermatogonia blocks spermatogenesis. Such animals are known as Klinefelter cats or cats suffering from Klinefelter syndrome.

Some male tortoiseshell cats with multiple cell lines, one of which has the normal male complement for a cat (i.e. 38,XY), have been fertile. An XY cell line is necessary for fertility but an XY cell line does not guarantee fertility.

The type of offspring that fertile male tortoiseshell cats produce will depend on whether or not the X chromosome in the 38,XY cell line is carrying the orange gene. If the cat is $38,X^oY$ then it will breed like a ginger tom (X^o means the X chromosome is carrying the orange gene). If it is $38,X^-Y$ (X^- means the X chromosome is not carrying the orange gene) the cat will breed like a black or tabby tom, depending upon which autosomal coat colour genes it has.

1. Fusion of placental blood vessels in multiple conceptions so that secretions from a male embryo can affect the development of a female twin embryo. This happens most commonly in cattle and the affected female is called a *freemartin* (Box 5.6).
2. Mutation of the Tdy gene or any one of the cascade of genes that are involved in sex differentiation. The animals usually develop as intersexes. This occurs most commonly in dogs, goats and pigs, and less commonly in horses (Box 5.7).
3. Mutation of an X-linked gene so that target organs cannot respond to the secretion of testosterone. The mutated gene is called 'the testicular feminisation gene' (Tfm). This is a rare mutation but it has been seen in a number of species (Box 5.8).
4. Abnormal number of X chromosomes. There can be an excess of X chromosomes, e.g. three X

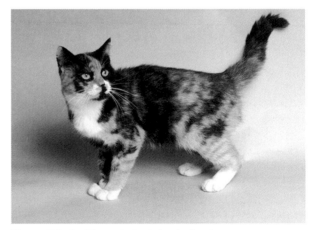

Figure 5.1 Fertile male tortoiseshell cat.

instead of two (triple X syndrome), or too few X chromosomes, i.e. XO (known as Turner syndrome after the person who first described it in humans). There may be a combination of these chromosome complements in the same animal, i.e. the animal is a mosaic or chimera.

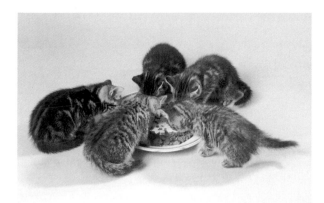

Figure 5.2 Five kittens from a litter sired by the male tortoiseshell cat pictured in Fig. 5.1. There were three males and two females. The females inherited the orange gene from the X chromosome of their father and were tortoiseshell.

This condition is seen most commonly in the horse (Box 5.9).

5. Abnormal number of X chromosomes together with a Y chromosome (XXY). This is called the Klinefelter syndrome. Affected animals are phenotypic males (because of the presence of the Y chromosome) but they are infertile because the presence of the two X chromosomes blocks spermatogenesis. It is recognised most commonly in the cat in association with the tortoiseshell coat colour but has been reported in a number of other species.

6. True hermaphrodites. Here the animal has both an ovary and a testis. It is difficult to understand how this development can occur! It is seen very rarely in our domestic animals but has been reported occasionally in the pig.

INTERSEXES (PSEUDOHERMAPHRODITES)

Intersexuality describes the condition whereby an animal has morphological aspects of both a male and a female (Box 5.10).

Intersexuality in the dog and cat

Intersexuality is more common in the dog than the cat. Intersex dogs usually present as females that do

---

Box 5.6 Freemartins

- Freemartins occur most commonly in cattle.
- They are infertile females born as twins with males.
- In cows carrying twins the blood vessels of the placenta of each fetus usually fuse (this is so in approximately 92% of pregnancies) so that the two fetuses have a common blood circulation.
- Thus, when the normal male twin starts to differentiate, all the secretions it produces also pass into the female fetus.
- Depending on when the placental fusion takes place the female twin will receive some Mullerian inhibition substance and some testosterone.
- The result is that the freemartin has an external phenotype of a female but has a short vagina (which is the posterior – caudal – vagina), no cervix, various degrees of inhibition of development of the uterine body, uterine horns and uterine tubes, and small, undifferentiated gonads.
- Another consequence of the fused placental blood vessels is that bone marrow precursor cells from the male and female mix so that the freemartin and her male twin have some blood cells that are genetically male (originating from the male fetus) and some blood cells that are genetically female (originating from the female). Thus their blood cells are chimeric and their chromosome complement is 60,XX/60XY. This phenomenon can be used in the newborn calf to diagnose placental fusion during pregnancy and so freemartinism.
- The condition is also seen occasionally in sheep, rarely in goats and very rarely in pigs. In the horse, freemartinism has not been confirmed because twins are not very often carried to term. The freemartin condition has not been diagnosed in cats and dogs but sex chromosome chimerism has.

---

not come into season. This is because the gonads do not develop properly and either remain undifferentiated or are ovo-testes, i.e. have some characteristics of both an ovary and a testis.

Box 5.7 Sex reversal in the horse

Some infertile 'mares' have been found to have a 64,XY normal male chromosome complement. These animals are, in fact, sex-reversed males. They do not have a normal Tdy gene and so the testes and hence the tubular genitalia of the male do not develop. Such animals have a female external phenotype; internally they have a uterus and either undifferentiated ovaries or ovaries with very little follicular development.

Box 5.8 Testicular feminisation

Testicular feminisation is caused by an X-linked gene (Tfm) that renders the target organs incapable of converting testosterone to dihydrotestosterone, which is the active hormone. Males carrying this gene on their X chromosome develop a testis, due to the action of the Tdy gene on the Y chromosome, the Sertoli cells secrete Mullerian inhibition substance and the development of the female ducts is suppressed as normal. The Leydig cells secrete testosterone but the Wolffian ducts are unable to respond and develop. Thus there are no tubular parts of the reproductive tract. In the absence of suppression there is an inbudding from the perineum to produce a vestibule and posterior (caudal) vagina. Therefore, the affected male develops as a phenotypic female with abdominal testes in an ovarian position. The gene does not seem to have any effect in the female and males always inherit the gene from their mother.

Box 5.9 Sex chromosome aneuploidy in the horse

Some infertile mares have been found to have sex chromosome aneuploidy (i.e. abnormal numbers of sex chromosomes). The most common is 63,XO (Turner's syndrome) and 63,XO/64,XX mixoploidy. Such animals are phenotypic females but usually do not come into season. Internally they have a uterus but small, undifferentiated ovaries. Other mares have had three X chromosomes, 65,XXX, and this is the triple X syndrome. These animals may cycle and some have even managed to breed but usually they are infertile because the XXX oogonium cannot undergo meiosis properly and produce normal ova.

Box 5.10 Terminology of intersexes

Hermaphrodites are animals that have an ovary and a testis. This is a very rare condition except in the pig. More commonly, animals have the phenotype of one sex but the gonads of the other. They were therefore called pseudohermaphrodites. In the past, intersexes were classified as male pseudohermaphrodites if they had a female external phenotype but gonads that were testicular, and female pseudohermaphrodites if they had a male phenotype but the gonads were ovarian. However, not all intersexes fall easily into these categories and so it is simpler to describe an animal just as an intersex.

The tubular genitalia do not develop normally – this can result in urinary problems. Urine from the bladder pools in a urogenital sinus instead of being expelled normally through a vagina and vestibule. The pooled urine acts as a source of bacterial multiplication and an ascending infection results. Less commonly, the urethra is narrower than normal and ascending infection may lead to the development of bladder stones. These can cause urethral blockage and the dog presents with urinary stasis.

Another complication is that in some intersex dogs the clitoris is enlarged; when the animal sits down it rubs on the ground and becomes sore. This causes the animal to lick the clitoris – making it even more painful.

Most intersex dogs are genetic females (78,XX) but have some male type characteristics. Thus there must have been a mutation in one of the cascade of genes that direct development towards the male phenotype.

Some are genetic males (78,XY). These may also have a female phenotype but some have male characteristics. Usually, the exact genetic basis of the intersexuality is not known. Nevertheless, there is one type of intersexuality in the cocker spaniel that is known to be due to an 'intersexuality' gene because the abnormality runs in particular lines or families of dogs.

Intersexuality in the cat seems to be rare. Male tortoiseshell cats are not really intersexes because they do not have any development of the female reproductive system.

Intersexuality in goats

Intersexuality in goats is caused by a recessive gene linked to the polling gene (the polling gene is a dominant gene that causes the absence of horns). The intersexuality gene disturbs the normal sex differentiation of genetic females.

- Females that are homozygous for the polling gene (PP,XX) are also homozygous for the intersexuality gene – and so are hornless and intersexes. Internally they have a uterus and testes-like gonads. Externally they have a basic female phenotype but there is an elongation of the anal–genital distance.
- Females that are heterozygous for the polling gene (Pp,XX) are heterozygous for the intersexuality gene. Since the polling gene is dominant such animals are hornless, but since the intersexuality gene is recessive, they are normal fertile females. However, they can pass on the intersexuality gene to their offspring.
- Males that are homozygous for the polling gene (PP,XY) are also homozygous for the intersexuality gene. However, the intersexuality gene

in the male does not usually have an effect. The animals are usually normal fertile, hornless males. They can, of course, pass on the intersexuality gene to their offspring. Occasionally, however, some PP,XY males have been infertile because the tubules in the caput epididymis are blocked.
- Males that are heterozygous for the polling gene (Pp,XY) are also heterozygous for the intersexuality gene. Such animals have always been normal, fertile hornless males.

Intersexuality in pigs

Intersexuality in pigs, like goats, is caused by an intersexuality gene. Unlike that in goats it has not been recognised as being linked to any other particular gene. Its effect is to cause abnormal development in a genetic female.

- Affected animals have a female external phenotype. Sometimes the clitoris is obviously enlarged, but not always.
- Internally affected animals have a uterus but the gonads are testes.
- Sometimes the testes descend into a scrotal position.
- Irrespective of whether the testes are abdominal or descended into a scrotum there is no spermatogenesis. This is because the animal is a genetic female (XX) and therefore does not have a spermatogenesis gene (which is on the Y chromosome). The intersexuality is due to a mutation in one of the cascade of genes that result in male phenotypic differentiation.

6

Blood groups and blood typing

Chapter contents

Core information: **Red blood cells have proteins on their cell surface coded for by genes. These proteins act as antigens and set up an antibody reaction when transfused into another animal. The different cell surface antigens constitute the blood groups. Animals have more complicated blood group systems than humans.**

Red blood cells (erythrocytes) have protein molecules on the surface of the cell that are antigenic (i.e. they stimulate an antibody reaction). The construction of these molecules is genetically determined. Different species have different genes, and different animals within a species have different alleles. Thus, different animals can have different red cell surface antigens. All the red cell surface antigens that arise from alleles at a single locus belong to the same blood group system.

- Allele A codes for antigen A, allele B codes for antigen B and allele O is what is called a 'null' allele in that it is a 'rubbish' allele and does not code for any molecule.
- The three alleles are co-dominant and so there are four possible blood groups in humans (Box 6.1).
- Humans are born with antibodies to 'foreign' red cells. They do not need to be challenged in

HUMAN BLOOD GROUPS

- Humans have the simplest system of red cell surface antigens.
- There is one gene locus and this locus has three alleles – A, B and O.

Box 6.1 Human ABO blood group system						
Genotype	AA	AB	AO	BB	BO	OO
Blood group	A	AB	A	B	B	O
Antigens	A	A & B	A	B	B	none

order for antibodies to be present. A person who is blood group A has anti-B antibodies circulating in the blood, and a person who is blood group B has anti-A antibodies. A person who is blood group AB has no antibodies to the red cell surface antigens. A person who is blood group O has anti-A and anti-B antibodies.

Determination of the blood group and blood type

The simplest method of determining the blood group of an individual is to challenge a sample of red blood cells with antibodies to red cell surface antigens. Each reagent should contain only one antibody and if there is a reaction then the red cells must carry that particular antigen. If the blood sample is challenged with reagents with antibodies to all the possible red cell surface antigens, the complete blood type can be determined.

The procedure is relatively simple for humans but blood types can be much more complicated in domestic animals (see below).

BLOOD TRANSFUSION REACTIONS

There are a number of unwanted clinical effects if a recipient is given the wrong blood:

- If blood from one individual is given to another without the blood of the donor matching the blood of the recipient then a *haemolytic reaction* will occur. Antibodies in the patient's blood lyse the red blood cells of the donor. Signs of such a reaction can be seen within minutes and include restlessness, incontinence, vocalisation, limb extension and opisthotonus.
- If whole blood is given, then the plasma of the donor will contain foreign plasma proteins and these will stimulate an *anaphylaxis*. The recipient's antibodies trigger mast cell degranulation and histamine release. Clinical signs will occur within minutes and include pruritus (itchiness), urticaria (redness) and bronchiospasm.
- Other blood components such as leucocytes and platelets are also antigenic – antibody response to these can cause a temperature rise of 0.5–1.0°C (1–2°F) and *pyrexia* (fever).

BLOOD GROUPS IN DOMESTIC ANIMALS

Domestic animals usually have much more complicated blood group systems than humans. Most species have more than one gene locus and each locus may have many different alleles.

Blood groups and blood transfusion in cats

The blood group system in the cat is the simplest of our domestic animals. There is one gene locus and three alleles – A and B and a rare AB allele. Cats can be type A, type B or type AB. Allele A is dominant to allele B, thus group B animals are homozygous for the B allele (i.e. B/B). The AB allele is recessive to allele A and co-dominant to allele B. The frequency of the different blood types depends upon geographic location and the breed of cat.

More than 95% of cats are group A, less than 5% are group B and less than 1% are AB. More than 98% of group B cats are pure-bred cats and the breeds with the highest frequency of group B are British Shorthair, Devon Rex and Cornish Rex. Cats are unusual compared with other domestic animals in that, like humans, they do have naturally occurring antibodies to other blood types.

All type B cats naturally have a high titre of anti-A antibodies. Therefore, it is very dangerous for type B cats to receive type A blood, and so it is important to accurately type the blood before any transfusion in order to avoid transfusion reactions (see above).

Fortunately, more than 95% of cats are type A and only about one-third of type A cats have circulating antibodies to type B cells (and these only weakly), so that the risk of a mismatched transfusion is low. There is now a commercial blood typing kit (RapidVet-H® feline) that can be used in the practice laboratory so that recipient and donor cats can always be matched.

The blood donor cat

There are a number of factors to consider before a cat can be accepted as a blood donor:

- Of course, blood donor cats need to be clinically healthy and free of blood-borne disease agents.

- They should have a packed cell volume (PCV) at the top of the normal range (normal = 25–40%) so that they are not more anaemic after collection than the treated animal.
- The maximum recommended donation volume is 10–12ml/kg body weight and so the donor cat should weigh more than 5kg.
- One unit of blood for cats is 50ml and collections are usually carried out every 4–6 weeks.
- The donor cat should be easily handled and remain unstressed by the collection procedure.

Blood groups and blood transfusion in dogs

In the dog, the red cell surface antigens are called 'dog erythrocyte antigens' which is abbreviated to DEAs. A total of 13 different blood groups have been described but antiserum for diagnosis is currently only available for five systems (Boxes 6.2, 6.3).

- For systems with just two alleles, dogs are either +ve or –ve for that system.
- In the DEA_1 system, only one of the four phenotypes is present in an individual animal. There is a linear dominance and 1.1 is the most dominant of the four alleles. Thus, a dog that is *phenotypically* $DEA_{1.1}$ +ve can have four possible *genotypes*, i.e. 1.1/1.1, or 1.1/1.2, or 1.1/1.3, or 1.1/–. A dog that is phenotypically $DEA_{1.2}$ +ve can have three possible genotypes, i.e. 1.2/1.2, or 1.2/1.3, or 1.2/– and so on.
- Some DEAs are more antigenic than others and therefore it is more important to ensure a match for these antigens when a blood transfusion is required.

- 98% of dogs are DEA_4 +ve and therefore these antigens will never be recognised as 'foreign'.
- 90% of dogs are positive for another DEA as well as DEA_4.
- Thus the least common blood type is DEA_4 +ve alone. These dogs are universal donors because their red blood cells will not be recognised as foreign by other dogs.
- The most common combinations with DEA_4 include either $DEA_{1.1}$ or $DEA_{1.2}$ and DEA_7.
- $DEA_{1.1}$ is particularly antigenic and if $DEA_{1.1}$ +ve blood is given to a $DEA_{1.1}$ –ve dog that has been sensitised, there will be a transfusion reaction.
- About 62% of dogs are DEA_1 +ve.

At birth, dogs do not naturally contain antibodies for the red cell surface antigens of all the foreign systems. Importantly, DEA_1 –ve dogs do not have naturally occurring antibodies for DEA_1. This means that, although this system is strongly antigenic, a single mismatched transfusion will not cause a problem.

Complete blood typing in the dog requires testing for all six of the possible blood groups. This would identify the rare, but useful, universal donor dogs. In practice this is rarely done. It is more common to identify $DEA_{1.1}$ –ve dogs so that these can be used as donors because it is these antigens that cause the main problems. There is a practice-based test available that will do this (Rapid Vet-H® canine). A second test is now also available that can differentiate $DEA_{1.1}$ +ve dogs from $DEA_{1.2}$ +ve dogs (ID-Card DEA_1).

The blood donor dog

The ideal donor would be an animal –ve for all except DEA_4. However, usually they are at least $DEA_{1.1}$ –ve.

Box 6.2 Blood group systems in the dog

Group	Number of alleles	Allele notation
DEA 1	4 (+?)	1.1, 1.2, 1.3 and null allele
DEA 3	2	3.0 and a null allele
DEA 4	2	4.0 and a null allele
DEA 5	2	5.0 and a null allele
DEA 7	2	6.0 and a null allele

Box 6.3 DEA_7

Strictly speaking the DEA_7 alleles do not code for a red cell surface antigen. More correctly they code for an antigen produced in tissue, which is then absorbed on to the red cells. However, thereafter they function like other red cell surface antigens.

- One unit of blood for the dog is 450ml.
- The dog should be over 25kg in weight since the donation volume is usually 16ml/kg.
- Frequency of donation is no more than once per month (1 donation/4 weeks)
- Ideally the donor should be over 1 year old and less than 8 years old.
- From a practical point of view they need to be easily handled and not resent collection from the jugular vein.
- They should be healthy and free from blood-borne diseases.

Blood groups in the horse

The horse blood group system is even more complicated than the dog. There are seven systems (i.e. gene loci) designated A, C, D, K, P, Q and U. The C, K and U systems each have one antigenic product and two alleles (including the null allele). The A, D, P and Q systems produce two or more antigens controlled by multiple alleles. Each antigen is designated by an upper case letter showing in which system it occurs, followed by a lower case letter for the individual antigen, e.g. Aa (Box 6.4).

As new populations of horses are studied new alleles are likely to be discovered:

- In some systems there are more alleles than antigens. Therefore some antigens are coded for by combinations of alleles.
- The two most potent antigens are A^a and Q^a. These are the antigens that are likely to be involved in isoerythrolysis in the horse (see below).
- The D group has the largest number of alleles and therefore is the most efficient group to be used in parentage analysis because unrelated animals will have different alleles.
- Naturally occurring antibodies to foreign blood are not usually present. Therefore one unmatched transfusion can occur between horses without any problems.
- The A^a antigen is very antigenic. Therefore an A^a –ve horse should not be given A^a +ve blood because it may stimulate anti-A^a antibodies in high titres even at the first transfusion and thus shorten the lifespan of the donor erythrocytes.
- Blood transfusion reactions are less likely when donor and recipient are closely related.
- Horses of different breeds are more likely to diverge and therefore transfusions between different breeds should be avoided unless blood tests are carried out.

Box 6.4 Blood group systems in the horse

System	No. of antigens	No. of alleles
A	7	12 – of which A^a is the one most clinically significant
C	1	2 – C^a and C^- (the latter is the null allele)
D	17	26 – including D^- (the null allele)
K	1	2 – K^a and K^- (the latter is the null allele)
P	4	8 – including P^- (the null allele)
Q	3	7 – of which Q^a is the one most clinically significant
U	1	2 – U^a and U^- (the latter is the null allele)

NEONATAL ISOERYTHROLYSIS

This is when red blood cells in the newborn undergo lysis in the body because of antibodies acquired from the dam. The condition arises because the fetus inherits red cell surface antigens from the sire that are absent in the dam. At parturition some of the neonatal red blood cells are absorbed and enter the circulation of the dam. The dam produces antibodies to these foreign red blood cells. Antibodies in the dam's blood get transferred to the offspring via the colostrum.

Usually, the first pregnancy does not cause problems in the offspring but this is when the dam is sensitised. Subsequent offspring receive high levels of antibody to their red blood cells when they suckle the colostrum. The result is that the offspring develops anaemia, jaundice and lethargy with raised pulse and respiration rate.

Neonatal isoerythrolysis in the cat

The condition is seen in B blood group cats that have been mated to A (or AB) group toms. The A group offspring will receive anti-A antibodies in the dam's colostrum which will be present whether or not there has been a previous pregnancy because B group cats always have anti-A antibodies in their blood which enter the colostrum. It would therefore be advisable to blood check toms to be mated to group B cats and either avoid using A group toms or, if they are used, artificially rear the kittens for the first 24–36 hours to avoid them receiving antibodies to their blood group in the colostrum.

Neonatal isoerythrolysis in the horse

The blood group alleles that cause the most problem in the horse are A^a and Q^a, and the most important is A^a (they are very immunogenic). When an A^a –ve dam is mated to an A^a +ve sire, the offspring may be A^a +ve. At parturition some of the foal's blood is absorbed by the dam and there is a rapid stimulation of anti-A^a antibodies. The antibody levels do not reach a high enough titre to cause a problem at the first parturition because colostrum is only absorbed in the first few hours after birth (approximately 16 hours). However, if there are subsequent A^a +ve foals then there will be high levels of anti A^a antibodies in the mare's colostrum immediately. The problem can be avoided in a number of ways:

- Only use A^a -ve sires with A^a –ve dams.
- Foals from mares that have already produced a foal with isoerythrolysis can be blood tested at birth. If the foal is A^a –ve then it is safe for them to suckle the dam.
- If the foal is A^a +ve then they should be removed from the dam and not allowed to suckle her for 36 hours after birth. During this time the foal can either be fostered on to an A^a +ve dam, given milk from an A^a +ve dam or fed artificial milk. After 36 hours there will be few antibodies in the dam's milk and furthermore the foal will not be able to absorb them in the stomach because the pH will have risen and the macromolecules will be broken down.

Neonatal isoerythrolysis in the dog

The DEA1.1 allele has been associated with neonatal erythrolysis in the dog. If DEA1.1 –ve bitches are mated to DEA1.1 +ve males they may produce DEA1.1 +ve puppies. If the bitch has been mated in this way before or has had a blood transfusion then she will have been sensitised to DEA1.1 antigens. Any DEA1.1 +ve puppies will receive anti-DEA1.1 antibodies in the colostrum and will show haemolytic anaemia 1–3 days later.

7

Inbreeding, cross breeding and heterosis

> **Core information: Inbreeding increases homozygosity and reveals recessive genes. This will fix characteristics and enable the offspring to 'breed true'. Cross breeding increases heterozygosity and masks recessive genes. For this reason the offspring are often 'better' than either parent. This is heterosis.**

Having discussed the action of genes at the nuclear and cellular level it is now time to consider what happens in the whole animal with the different systems of breeding that man has imposed.

INBREEDING

Inbreeding is defined as breeding between related individuals. The results of inbreeding are:

- Reduction of heterozygosity and increase in homozygosity.
- The increase in homozygosity reveals recessive genes.
- The increase in homozygosity fixes genes and so animals are more likely to 'breed true'.

Relatives are more likely to have some alleles that are the same compared to non-related animals because relatives could have inherited the same allele from the same ancestor. When an animal

receives the same allele from its mother as from its father It means that the same allele is present on each of the two chromosomes carrying that gene locus. Therefore, *inbreeding increases homozygosity*.

Recessive alleles in the genome are only expressed when they occur in the homozygous state. Therefore, *inbreeding reveals* the presence of *recessive genes* because they are expressed in the phenotype.

When an animal is homozygous at a gene locus it has two copies of the same allele to pass on at that locus. Therefore, *inbreeding fixes the characteristic* and allows the animal *to breed true*.

Inbreeding is carried out when breeders are selecting for a particular characteristic and want to fix that characteristic in future populations. However, inbreeding is generally considered to be bad – why should this be? It is because inbreeding will reveal recessive alleles and 'bad' genes are often recessive (Box 7.1).

It is important to remember that inbreeding increases homozygosity for any gene, regardless of

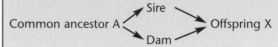
whether the gene has a beneficial effect on the fitness of the animal or whether it is deleterious. The chances of fixing 'good' genes are exactly the same as the chances of fixing 'bad' genes.

All animals carry *some* recessive genes that, in the homozygous state, would reduce viability and therefore could be considered as 'bad'. However, unrelated individuals usually have *different* 'bad' genes and so their offspring are not homozygous for any of them. Related individuals are more likely to have the same genes, 'good' or 'bad', and so their offspring are more likely to be homozygous for these good and bad genes.

What affects the outcome of inbreeding?

- The degree of relationship of the animals. The more closely related the animals, the more likely they are to have the same alleles (Boxes 7.2, 7.3).
- How many 'bad' alleles the related animals have in their genome. This will not be known because we never know all the alleles in an individual. Every animal will be carrying *some* undesirable alleles. Mating two related animals with very few

'bad' alleles is less likely to cause problems than mating related animals with many 'bad' alleles.
- Whether related animals have the *same* 'bad' alleles. Related animals are more likely to have more similar 'bad' alleles than unrelated animals. We can calculate the chances that offspring of related animals will be homozygous for a gene of whatever kind (Boxes 7.4, 7.5).

It can be seen from Box 7.5 that when brother and sister matings take place the chances of homozygosity at any one gene locus is 1 in 4 (that is what the 25% means). In other words this is very high – so it is not surprising that if there are bad genes within a family, such matings will reveal them. The less the relationship, the less are the chances of homozygosity at any locus.

Box 7.4 Coefficient of inbreeding

There is a mathematical expression that predicts the chances of homozygosity in the offspring due to the fact that the parents are related. This is called the coefficient of inbreeding and is defined as the probability of homozygosity at any locus in the offspring due to the fact that the parents had a common ancestor. The mathematical equation is:

$$F_x = (^1/_2)^{n-1} \times (1 + F_a)$$

where F_x = the coefficient of inbreeding of individual X, n = the number of arrows connecting the individual through the common ancestor, F_a = The coefficient of inbreeding of the common ancestor.

Box 7.5 Some examples of coefficients of inbreeding*

Full sibs	25%
Half sibs	12.5%
First cousins	6.35%
Grandparent/grandchild	12.5%

*The probability that any one gene will be homozygous by descent (it is assumed that the common ancestor is not inbred, i.e. $F_a = 0$).

Reasons for inbreeding

- The most common reason for inbreeding is to fix a characteristic that is desirable. What the breeder is in fact doing is hoping that the desirable gene will be fixed and not the undesirable one. It is really like Russian roulette!
- Sometimes inbreeding is deliberately carried out with the intention of detecting whether one of the parents is a carrier of a recessive gene (see chapter 3). How ethical this is will depend upon the gene involved. In the UK the deliberate production of a homozygous recessive animal that is deformed or ill can only be done under licence from the Home Office. The testing for something like coat colour does not need such strict control.

- Some laboratory animals, such as mice, are deliberately inbred so that lines of animals are genetically the same. This is essential for some genetic investigations and is always done under licence from the Home Office.

Inbreeding depression

This is an expression that describes the general reduction in vitality and viability of many inbred animals. It occurs because of the increase in homozygosity and therefore expression of recessive genes that are deleterious. It is most marked in characteristics such as fertility and progeny survivability. It is the main reason why inbreeding is generally considered to be a bad thing.

Line breeding

Line breeding is a form of inbreeding. It describes the practice of using an individual (e.g. a show champion) more than once in a pedigree. If an ancestor occurs several times in a pedigree the relationship (i.e. the proportion of genes that are likely to be the same) between the individual and the ancestor can be quite high.

When breeders carry out line breeding, what they are attempting to do is to make their animals as genetically similar to the champion ancestor as possible. However, since line breeding is a form of inbreeding, line breeding will also create inbreeding depression with a reduction in fertility and viability.

CROSS BREEDING

Cross breeding is defined as the breeding of unrelated individuals. The effects of crossing breeding are the opposite of inbreeding:

- increasing heterozygosity
- masking of recessive genes
- reducing the likelihood of breeding true.

Unrelated individuals, even if they are themselves inbred, are not likely to have the same alleles as each other and so their offspring will be heterozygous at many loci. Compared to the parent population therefore there will be an *increase in heterozygosity*.

When there is heterozygosity at a gene locus, no recessive gene will be expressed and so its presence will be masked. An animal that is heterozygous at a number of loci will produce a large variety of gametes (because there will be a variety of combinations of alleles) and so they are less likely to breed true (i.e. produce offspring that are very like themselves).

The effects of cross breeding are particularly noticeable on such traits as fertility and viability of offspring. Hence there is said to be an 'increase in vigour' – hybrid vigour or heterosis.

Hybrid vigour (heterosis)

Hybrid vigour (heterosis) arises because of the masking of recessive genes, which depress viability in the homozygous state. Animals with hybrid vigour have a superior performance compared to their parents. Hybrid vigour is seen most obviously when two inbred (but different) lines of animals are mated. Each inbred line will be showing inbreeding depression because of homozygosity for different genes. Their offspring will be heterozygous for all those genes and therefore the deleterious recessive genes will be masked – and so the offspring will show increased vigour.

8

Selection and eradication schemes

Core information: **To choose which animals to breed from we need to know which of their characteristics are produced by genes since only these will be passed to the next generation. A performance test is useful for characteristics that are governed by dominant or co-dominant genes because then the phenotype reflects the genotype. Pedigree analysis and evaluation of siblings will give an indication of what genes an animal is carrying because relatives have similar genes. However, this is not a 100% accurate prediction. A more accurate way of testing what genes an animal is carrying is to carry out test matings and evaluate the offspring. This is a progeny test. BVA/Kennel club schemes to eradicate eye defects and hip and elbow dysplasias are performance tests, as is the FAB scheme for polycystic disease in cats. New methods of molecular genetic examination are allowing the identification of carriers of recessive genes without the necessity of carrying out test matings.**

The different breeds in our domestic animals have been developed through selective breeding by man. This selective breeding has involved inbreeding in order to fix desired characteristics (i.e. to create homozygosity) and it has therefore also created homozygosity for undesirable characteristics that were also within the original genotype. Some undesirable characteristics can be fairly innocuous, for example an unwanted coat colour, but some are a danger to the health and welfare of the individual animal.

New mutations also occur. Some of these mutations have resulted in traits that man has considered desirable, for example the absence of top-coat fur in Rex cats, but some have compromised the health of the animals.

Breeders are now trying to remove genes that cause anomalies from their breeding lines. This can be difficult to do. For example:

- If there is a breed with a small number of animals and the gene is present in a large proportion of the breed, then culling all carriers of a deleterious gene will severely deplete the breed numbers. This will reduce the gene pool and the amount of genetic variation within the breed.
- When we try to improve a breed or line we are selecting *for* some characteristics and *against* others. If the genes governing the characteristics we want are *linked* to characteristics we do not want, then it is very difficult indeed to make any improvement.
- In addition, using only a few animals to produce the next generation will increase inbreeding, which results in an increased homozygosity and inbreeding depression. As we have seen, one of the results of inbreeding depression is reduced fertility!

METHODS OF SELECTION

There are a number of different ways to choose which animals will be the dams and sires of the next generation (Box 8.1).

Performance test

The simplest method of selection is based upon the phenotype or performance of the animal. Therefore it is called a *performance test*. This selection method is best for characteristics that are governed by single genes and is most efficient for dominant genes. Any animal carrying a dominant gene, whether in the heterozygous or homozygous state, will express that gene and so it is fairly easy to remove unwanted dominant genes from the population simply by not breeding from affected animals. It is more difficult to eliminate recessive genes because carrier animals cannot be detected by their phenotype or performance.

The British Veterinary Association (BVA)/Kennel Club/ International Sheep Dog Society scheme for the eradication of inherited eye diseases and the British Veterinary Association/Kennel Club hip dysplasia and elbow dysplasia eradication schemes are performance tests. The phenotype of the animal is examined and an assessment made as to whether the animal is carrying genes for the anomaly.

Limitations of performance testing
Recessive genes
Selection by means of phenotype does not work so well for anomalies produced by recessive genes. This is because the phenotype only reveals the presence of the recessive genes if they are in the homozygous state. If only the affected (homozygous) animals are culled (because they are the ones that can be identified) the gene frequency will be reduced but the gene cannot be completely eliminated unless heterozygous carrier animals can be detected and eliminated. Most of the inherited eye defects in dogs are controlled by recessive genes. Thus eradication schemes are removing the homozygous animals from the breeding population but not the heterozygotes.

Polygenic and multifactorial characteristics
Polygenic traits are caused by a number of genes and multifactorial traits are caused by the interaction of genes and the environment. It is extremely difficult to eliminate such conditions just by looking at the phenotype of the animal. An apparently normal animal could quite well be carrying *some* of the deleterious genes. Unfortunately both hip dysplasia and elbow dysplasia in the dog are polygenic, multifactorial conditions. This is one of the reasons that although eradication schemes have been running for a number of years we still see the clinical condition in dogs.

Box 8.1 Selection methods

- Performance testing
- Progeny testing
- Pedigree analysis and ancestor evaluation
- Performance testing of siblings (brothers and sisters)
- Molecular genetic screening

Age of onset of gene expression

If the gene is expressed only after the animal is old enough to have started to breed then it can take longer to eradicate the problem because some genes will be passed to the next generation before they are expressed in the parents. This is the situation in some inherited eye defects in dogs. The animals can be examined when young and appear to be free of the anomaly and yet develop the anomaly later in life. Thus it is difficult to select animals to produce the next generation of animals.

Progeny testing

One way of checking whether an animal is a carrier of a recessive gene is to perform the back cross to the recessive (see Chapter 3). In other words, a mating is carried out and the offspring (progeny) are examined (tested). This is therefore called a *progeny test*. It is useful for revealing carriers of a recessive gene and also for identifying genes responsible for sex-limited characteristics (Box 8.2).

Limitations of progeny testing
Breeding from animals with an anomaly
Checking for a carrier of a recessive gene by means of the back cross to the recessive involves crossing to known homozygous or known heterozygous animals. In the situation where the cross is designed to identify carriers of a gene that produces an anomaly, the homozygous animal

---

Box 8.2 Identification of sex-limited genes by a progeny test

Some genes are only expressed in one sex even though both sexes carry genes for the characteristic. The best example of this is the genes responsible for milk yield. Both the male and female carry genes that control yield, protein content and butter fat of milk but these genes are only expressed in the female. Therefore, to check what milk genes the male is carrying, he has to be mated and the milk yield of his daughters evaluated. Half of the daughter's milk genes will come from the father, thus his milk genes can be assessed.

---

may not be able to breed or may be clinically unsuitable for breeding. In such a situation only a backcross to the heterozygote would be used. Even this cross should only be done under strict control because the deliberate production of anomalous animals is not something to be contemplated lightly.

Lethal genes
Lethal genes are those that result in the death of the embryo *in utero*. Therefore, it is not possible to check for carriers of such genes by looking for affected progeny, because they are never born. If such crosses were to be carried out the embryos would have to be examined either by laparotomy or killing the mother. Alternatively, one could assume that abnormally low litter sizes were due to embryonic death as a result of homozygosity for a lethal gene. The classic example of a lethal gene is the Manx gene in cats, which is lethal in the homozygous state.

Pedigree analysis and ancestor evaluation

It would be possible to select against a particular anomaly by looking at an individual's pedigree. If the anomaly has appeared in the ancestors of the animal then there is a chance that the individual has inherited the gene causing the anomaly. One could then choose to avoid breeding from this family or line. The drawback to this system is that not all animals whose ancestors are affected will have inherited the deleterious gene. Thus, failure to breed from the line could mean that many good genes would be going to waste.

Performance testing of siblings

Brothers and sisters (full siblings) can be used to gauge the chances of each other having genes for a particular anomaly. Full sibs have 50% of their genes that are the same – if one animal in a litter has the abnormality there is a high chance that the apparently normal siblings will be carriers of recessive allele. To avoid passing on the allele one could refrain from breeding from littermates of affected animals. However, once again, not all the unaffected siblings will be carriers of the recessive allele and so culling all littermates may mean that some good genes are being lost (Box 8.3). Gauging the performance of full brothers and sisters can be a protracted exercise if the animal normally only produces one offspring at a time (e.g. the horse). To speed things up it is possible to compare the offspring of one male mated to a number of different females. These offspring will be *half sibs*. Half sibs do not have as many genes in common as full sibs and so the accuracy of the test is reduced.

Molecular genetic screening

Recent advances in molecular genetics mean that it is now possible to identify certain individual genes in an animal's genome. DNA testing is usually more sensitive, and often much quicker, than other forms of tests. There are two broad categories of gene testing:

- In certain conditions the gene that causes the anomaly has been identified and sequenced. In this case it is possible to test for the gene itself. This is called a *gene probe*.
- In other conditions the exact gene is not known, but it is known that it is always linked either to another gene or to a certain DNA sequence. Thus, either the linked gene or the linked DNA sequence can be identified. In this case *marker DNA* is used.

An important tool in the molecular analysis of animals is the polymerase chain reaction (PCR). This reaction creates millions of copies of the sample of DNA. Thus even very small samples of DNA can be used for analysis.

By means of molecular genetic techniques the animal can be classified as clear, heterozygous or homozygous for the undesired gene. Using this information, breeding programmes can be constructed so that the unwanted gene is removed from the population without culling too many animals. This lessens the risk of reducing the gene pool to such an extent that other, more serious, recessive genes are revealed. A gene test is only really useful for conditions caused by single genes. At the moment it is not possible to test for polygenic conditions such as hip dysplasia.

It is now possible to test for a number of inherited conditions in the dog by molecular genetic methods. Molecular genetic testing in the cat is less advanced. However, new tests are being developed. Polycystic kidney disease in the cat, which is caused by a single autosomal dominant gene, is currently tested for using the principles of performance testing but a new gene test is being developed; if validated, it will be introduced for routine use (Box 8.4).

BVA/KENNEL CLUB HIP DYSPLASIA SCHEME

Hip dysplasia is a polygenic, multifactorial condition of the hips. Clinically there is a variable degree of malformation of both the femoral head and acetabulum of the hip, which results in

---

Box 8.3 Chances of littermates of an affected animal being carriers of a recessive gene

There is a two in three chance that apparently normal individuals are a carrier of a recessive if they are littermates of homozygous recessive animals, i.e. 66%. This is fairly easy to work out from a punnet square. If the individual homozygous for a recessive gene has phenotypically normal parents they both must be heterozygous carriers, for example:

Parents:	$Bb \times Bb$
Gametes:	$B + b\ B + b$
Offspring:	$BB + Bb + Bb + bb$
Phenotypically normal:	$BB + Bb + Bb$

Ratio of carriers:normal in phenotypically normal: 2:1 (i.e. 66%)

Box 8.4 Eradication schemes

- British Veterinary Association/Kennel Club hip dysplasia scheme
- British Veterinary Association/Kennel Club elbow dysplasia scheme
- British Veterinary Association/Kennel Club/International sheep dog society eye scheme
- Polycystic kidney disease scheme

lameness, pain and reactive arthritic changes. It is a particular problem in certain breeds of dogs. The condition is exacerbated by increased exercise and good feeding, leading to rapid growth in the young prepubescent animal.

The eradication scheme started in June 1978 for German shepherd dogs and for other breeds in 1983. The basis of the scheme is radiographic examination of young adult animals in order to identify signs of malformation. For most breeds the examination takes place after the animal is 12 months old but for giant breeds it is delayed until they are 18 months old.

The radiographs are taken by the clients' own veterinary surgeon and these are then interpreted by a panel of experts. It is very important for accurate interpretation that the radiographs are taken with the animal in the correct position. The animal is placed with its back on the x-ray plate with the legs equally extended, adducted and inwardly rotated (Box 8.5).

A number of parameters are assessed on each hip by a member of the panel of experts and each parameter is given a score. The total for each examined point is the hip 'score'. The lowest score, 0, indicates normality and the highest score, 106, indicates the worst possible expression of hip dysplasia.

The names of Kennel Club registered dogs scored under the scheme, together with the scores, are sent to the Kennel Club for publication and inclusion on the animals' documents (results of dogs not registered with the Kennel Club will not be sent on). Over the years a number of dogs have been examined from each breed and so it is possible to calculate a 'breed mean score' (BMS) for hip dysplasia. The breeds are classified into six groups (A–F) based on the number of animals in the breed that have been examined (Table 8.1). The BMS for breeds in which a high number of animals have been examined is more significant than in a breed in which only a few animals have been examined.

The recommendation after the examination of the hips is that only animals with a score well below the breed mean score should be used for breeding purposes – the BVA informs the Kennel Club of registered dogs with a score of 8 or less and no more than 6 on either hip. By following these recommendations the aim is slowly to reduce the

> **Box 8.5** Positioning for radiography of the hip for submission to the hip dysplasia scheme
>
> ■ The dog should be placed on its back with the pelvis in the middle of the cassette and the x-ray beam centred on the midline between the hips (i.e. the centring point should be at the level of the cranial edge of the pubis).
> ■ In order to avoid rotation, the head and body should be supported in a straight line by a cradle or by blocks at the thorax. Tilting of any part of the dog's body is likely to cause axial rotation of the pelvis and asymmetry of the hips.
> ■ The hind legs should be *fully* extended and adducted so that the femora lie parallel to each other and parallel to the film.
> ■ The legs should be inwardly rotated so that the patellae lie centrally in the trochlear grooves.
> ■ Suitable ties or tape should be used to achieve correct adduction and inward rotation – poor positioning which allows either lateral or longitudinal tilt of the pelvis may prevent accurate radiological assessment of the hips.
> ■ If the radiograph shows axial rotation of the pelvis, this may be corrected by raising the hip on the side on which the image of the obturator foramen is smaller.

Table 8.1 BVA/Kennel Club breed groups*

Group	No. animals examined	No. breeds in group
A	>1000	22
B	500–999	13
C	100–499	32
D	40–99	12
E	10–32	33
F	<10	No data

*BVA data as at 10.10.01

BMS. The genes responsible for the condition will then be eliminated from the breed (Table 8.2).

There is a problem with this approach. This is a performance test and selection on the basis of phenotype is not very efficient for polygenic multifactorial conditions. By removing affected

Table 8.2 Breeds with the highest breed mean scores for hip dysplasia*

Breed	No. examined	Score range	BMS
Otterhound	114	4–102	43
Clumber Spaniel	469	0–102	42
Sussex Spaniel	105	7–101	37
Bullmastiff	610	0–104	28
Newfoundland	2784	0–106	28
Gordon Setter	1719	0–104	25
St Bernard	247	0–73	23
Briard	635	0–99	20
Old English Sheepdog	1276	0–100	20
English Setter	2021	0–95	19
Golden Retriever	23,746	0–106	19
Welsh Springer Spaniel	1045	0–104	19
German Shepherd Dog	31,654	0–106	19

*BVA data as at 10.10.01

individuals from the breeding population we are removing some 'bad' genes. However, in polygenic conditions, normal or only slightly affected animals may still be carrying 'bad' genes but they can be masked by other so-called 'minor' genes. Furthermore, with conditions that are affected by the 'environment', e.g. nutrition and exercise, the condition can be masked by the environment. For example, a dog with hip dysplasia genes that has rapid growth and heavy exercise when young will show the condition more than a similar dog which has had slow growth and little exercise at a young age.

BVA/KENNEL CLUB ELBOW DYSPLASIA SCHEME

Elbow dysplasia is the abnormal development of the cartilage of the elbow joint. The resultant wear leads to secondary osteoarthritic changes and lameness. In the dog there are three primary lesions:

- osteochondritis dissecans (OCD)
- fragmented or ununited coronoid process (FCP)
- ununited anconeal process (UAP).

Like hip dysplasia, the condition is caused by a number of genes (i.e. it is polygenic) and is also influenced by environmental factors such as growth rate, diet and exercise (i.e. it is mutifactorial).

The eradication scheme was started in 1998 and is conducted in a similar manner to that of the hip dysplasia scheme. Currently two views of the elbow joint are required – extended lateral and flexed lateral (previously a craniocaudal view was also needed but this requirement was dropped in January 2004). The clients' own veterinary surgeon takes the radiographs when the animal is one or more years old and these are examined by a panel of experts. Each elbow is graded on a 0–3 scale, with 0 indicating normality and 3 severe elbow dysplasia.

The names of Kennel Club registered dogs graded under the scheme, together with the results, are sent to the Kennel Club for publication and inclusion on the relevant documents (details and results of dogs not registered with the Kennel Club will not be sent on).

Not all animals with signs of elbow dysplasia will be lame. This is the subclinical population and has been likened to the part of an iceberg that is submerged! It is recommended that only animals with a grade of 0 or 1 be used for breeding (Boxes 8.6, 8.7).

BVA/KENNEL CLUB/INTERNATIONAL SHEEP DOG SOCIETY EYE SCHEME

This is the oldest eradication scheme in the UK, having been established for more than 30 years. It

Box 8.6 Grading scheme for elbow dysplasia

Grade	Description
0	Normal
1	Mild ED
2	Moderate ED or primary lesion
3	Severe ED

Box 8.7 Breeds with a high incidence of elbow dysplasia

Basset Hound	Bernese Mountain Dog
English Mastiff	German Shepherd
Golden Retriever	Great Dane
Irish Wolfhound	Labrador Retriever
Newfoundland	Rottweiler

Box 8.8 Conditions covered by the BVA/KC/ISDS eye scheme

Goniodysgenesis/primary glaucoma
Persistent papillary membrane
Persistent hyperplastic primary vitreous
Retinal dysplasia
Collie eye anomaly
Hereditary cataract
Primary lens luxation
Generalised progressive retinal atrophy
Central retinal atrophy

is a performance test like the hip and elbow dysplasia schemes. Animals are examined and assessed to see whether they are suffering from the disease (and therefore homozygous for the condition, since most of the problems are caused by recessive genes). The scheme currently covers nine hereditary eye conditions in 47 different breeds.

The causal gene and mode of inheritance of an anomaly can be different in different breeds – it is beyond the scope of this text to go into the detail of each. Interpretation of the morphology of the eye and its structures is very complex so all the examinations are carried out by veterinary specialists in ophthalmology. These specialists comprise the Eye Panel Working Party (Box 8.8).

The breeds and conditions are divided into Schedule 1 and Schedule 3. Schedule 1 lists the known inherited eye diseases in the breeds where there is enough scientific information to show that the condition is inherited in that breed – and often what is the mode of inheritance. For the breeds in Schedule 1 a certificate is issued with results of 'affected' or 'unaffected' – these results are recorded and published by the Kennel Club. Schedule 3 lists those breeds in which the conditions are only suspected as hereditary and therefore are 'under investigation'. With further work, breeds and conditions in Schedule 3 may be confirmed as inherited and therefore moved to Schedule 1.

Dogs are best first examined before they are one year old – thereafter an annual examination will reveal any later developing anomalies. Since some conditions are congenital, i.e. present at birth, recognition of some conditions requires examination of very young puppies between 6–12 weeks and so litter screening is also carried out in some circumstances.

FELINE ADVISORY BUREAU (FAB) POLYCYSTIC KIDNEY DISEASE SCREENING SCHEME

Polycystic kidney disease (PKD) is caused by a single autosomal dominant gene, so every animal carrying even a single copy of the gene will show clinical signs. Homozygosity for the gene causes such gross abnormal development of the kidneys that there is prenatal death – this is another example of a lethal gene (Box 8.9).

The screening programme is based on ultrasonographic examination of the kidney by a veterinary specialist. The cats should be over 10 months old in order that, when no cysts are found, there is confidence that small cysts have not been missed. A copy of the result of the scan is sent to the FAB. By the end of 2004 about 2000 cats in Britain had been screened.

Recently the Veterinary Genetics Laboratory (VGL) in California has developed a gene test to identify cats that carry the gene for polycystic

---

Box 8.9 Polycystic kidney disease

The disease was first reported in 1967 but the condition has been more of a problem in the last 10 years. It is particularly common in Persian cats. Worldwide approximately one-third of Persian cats are affected. The gene has now been introduced into other breeds, such as Burmillas and exotic shorthairs, which have been developed using the Persian bloodline.

Affected animals have multiple cysts within the kidneys. These cysts may be small at first but they grow larger in time and severely disrupt the ability of the kidney to function – affected cats develop kidney failure. The rate of progression of the clinical disease is very variable and the onset of renal failure may be anywhere between two and ten years.

Box 8.10 Diseases and breeds for which molecular testing is available

Canine leukocyte adhesion deficiency	Irish Setter
Progressive retinal atrophy	Irish Setter & Miniature Long-haired Dachshund
Von Willebrand's disease	Irish Red and White Setter
Copper toxicosis	Bedlington Terriers
Fucosidosis	English Springer Spaniels
Phosphofructokinase deficiency	English Springer Spaniels
Congenital stationary night blindness	Briards
Globoid cell leucodystrophy	West Highland White Terriers
Pyruvate kinase deficiency	West Highland White Terriers

---

kidney disease. If this new gene test proves to be accurate, then it is likely that it will supersede the FAB ultrasonographic screening scheme. To date the test has been used in a relatively small number of cats from the USA.

MOLECULAR GENETIC SCREENING

Molecular genetic screening is the laboratory detection of a particular gene in a sample of DNA. It is also known as DNA testing. The techniques can detect carriers of defective genes (heterozygotes) as well as homozygotes, so they are particularly useful for the eradication of recessive genes (Box 8.10).

In the UK the Animal Health Trust is offering a commercial service and will carry out molecular genetic screening for a number of diseases in the dog. A molecular genetic test is also being developed for polycystic kidney disease in cats. The same condition may be caused by a different gene in different breeds, so a test for one breed is not necessarily applicable to another.

Canine leukocyte adhesion deficiency

Canine leukocyte adhesion deficiency (CLAD) is a disease of the immune system found in Irish Setters. The gene responsible has an autosomal recessive mode of inheritance. The Animal Health Trust's test probes directly for the gene in DNA from a blood sample. It diagnoses Irish Setters affected with this disease and also those dogs that are carriers. DNA testing for CLAD is carried out under a screening scheme run with the Kennel Club (results are made available through the Kennel Club Website).

Congenital stationary night blindness in Briards

Congenital stationary night blindness (CSNB) (also called hereditary retinal dystrophy) in Briards is caused by an autosomal recessive gene. The symptoms include night blindness and a loss of vision in daylight that can vary between individual dogs. The Animal Health Trust's test probes directly for the gene and distinguishes affected, carrier and normal individuals. The test can be carried out on material from the buccal mucosa.

Copper toxicosis in Bedlington Terriers

Copper toxicosis is a hereditary disease in which failure in the ability of the liver to expel dietary copper leads to a build-up in the liver, causing illness and death. It is inherited as an autosomal recessive gene. The test is based upon the fact that *marker DNA* (known as a DNA microsatellite) is situated near to the defective gene and will be inherited along with the disease. (The marker is not part of the disease gene and so the test works in a different way from tests where the genetic defect itself is detected, e.g. progressive retinal atrophy in the Irish Setter.) For each dog tested, 3–5 generation pedigrees with disease status indicated are also requested. That way, as more data are collected the test can be refined. At present the test has an accuracy of up to 95%. Submitted samples can be either buccal mucosa or peripheral blood. Results are kept on a database and made available to the Bedlington Terrier Association.

Fucosidosis in English Springer Spaniels

The genetic defect underlying fucosidosis in English Springer Spaniels is a deletion (i.e. a small segment of DNA is missing) within the fucosidase gene. Fucosidase is an enzyme necessary for the normal activity and function of nerves. The test can distinguish between normal, carrier and affected dogs. It works by using the polymerase chain reaction to amplify the region of the gene that spans the deletion and then separating the DNA fragments on the basis of their size. The DNA fragment from the disease gene can be recognised because it is smaller than that from the normal gene. The test is carried out on DNA from a blood sample.

Phosphofructokinase deficiency in English Springer Spaniels

Deficiency of the enzyme phosphofructokinase leads to haemolytic anaemia and jaundice after exercise. The genetic defect underlying phospho-fructokinase deficiency in English Springer Spaniels is a small change (i.e. point mutation) in the phosphofructokinase gene. The DNA test involves determining the structure of the gene in the critical region using the polymerase chain reaction. This disorder shows an autosomal recessive mode of inheritance. It has also been found in the American

Cocker Spaniel. The test is carried out on DNA from a blood sample.

Progressive retinal atrophy (PRA) in Miniature Long-haired Dachshunds

PRA is a term for retinal degenerations occurring in many breeds of dog. Many forms of PRA exist, each form being confined to one or a few breeds only. The disease results in a degeneration of the retina resulting in loss of vision, and often leading to blindness. The disease in Miniature Long-haired Dachshunds is caused by a mutation to a gene involved in sight that has now been identified. The test can be carried out either on DNA from blood or buccal mucosa.

Progressive retinal atrophy in Irish Setters

PRA in the Irish Setter leads to night-blindness and eventually total blindness. Symptoms can occur as early as 6 weeks of age. The gene responsible has been identified and has an autosomal recessive mode of inheritance. The Animal Health Trust's test probes directly for the gene and can be done on a blood sample. It provides definitive information on the genetic status of this disease. DNA testing for PRA in Irish setters is carried out under a screening scheme run with the Kennel Club. Results are made available through the Kennel Club website.

Pyruvate kinase deficiency in West Highland White Terriers

This disease results in a deficiency of the enzyme in red blood cells. The clinical signs include severe haemolytic anaemia and disorders of the bone marrow and the liver. The condition is due to a deletion of a small segment of DNA within the gene – the mutated gene has an autosomal recessive mode of inheritance. The Animal Health Trust's test probes for the gene itself. It diagnoses which West Highland White Terriers are affected with this disease and also those dogs that are carriers. The test can be carried out on DNA from a blood sample.

9

Reproductive physiology

Chapter contents

Core information: Reproduction in the male and female is governed by gonadotropin releasing hormone (GnRH) produced by the hypothalamus, a part of the brain. This directs the anterior pituitary, which secretes follicle stimulating hormone (FSH) and luteinising hormone (LH). These secretions control the gonads (ovaries and testes). In the female, FSH stimulates the growth of follicles, which produce oestrogen. LH causes ovulation and the formation of the corpus luteum from the collapsed follicle after ovulation. The corpus luteum secretes progesterone. Progesterone is the hormone that maintains pregnancy. In the male, LH stimulates the interstitial cells (Leydig cells) of the testis to produce testosterone. FSH stimulates the Sertoli cells in the testis to produce androgen-binding hormone, which stimulates spermatogenesis. Parturition is triggered by corticosterolds from the fetus. These start a cascade of events in the dam leading to expulsion of the fetus. Milk production is stimulated by prolactin, which is produced in the anterior pituitary. In both the male and the female the levels of each hormone are controlled by a seesaw-like feedback mechanism that maintains equilibrium.

Genetic material is in the nucleus of each cell of the body. However, the genes can only be passed on to the next generation via the gametes, i.e. the ova in the female and the spermatozoa in the male.

The genetic sex of an animal is established at fertilisation depending upon whether the spermatozoon contains an X or Y chromosome. The phenotype of the animal not only depends upon the action of the sex-determining genes, which trigger gonadal development, but also on the secretion of reproductive hormones from the gonads. It is the action of these hormones that eventually leads to the development of the reproductive system. The reproductive hormones control ovulation and fertilisation, implantation and growth of the embryo into a fetus, and eventually parturition. The production of new reproductively competent individuals relies on the production of the reproductive hormones at the appropriate level at the appropriate time. This section of the book examines male and female reproductive physiology in general and then discusses the different species in more detail.

The principles of reproductive physiology are the same in the different species. Control starts in the brain. The system is governed by the part of the brain called the *hypothalamus*. The hypothalamus sends signals to the *pituitary* gland. An alternative name for the pituitary gland is the *hypophysis* or *hypophyseal gland*. The pituitary gland controls the gonads (testes or ovaries) and these in turn influence other parts of the reproductive tract via their hormones (Fig. 9.1).

In the male, the reproductive hormones control:

■ the production of spermatozoa in the testis
■ the development of the male type phenotype (for example, the thickened cheek pouches of the tom cat and the crest or curve of the neck in the stallion)
■ the development of the male libido.

In the female, reproductive hormones control:
■ the development of the follicles and maturation of the oocytes (also called ova or eggs)
■ the maintenance of pregnancy and lactation
■ the development of female behaviour.

In the male there is a simple 'seesaw' system of positive and negative feedback mechanisms between the testes, the anterior pituitary and the hypothalamus so that equilibrium is maintained. In the female, there is a more complex system of interrelated cycles that allow for the production of ova without fertilisation, and also pregnancy and lactation.

HYPOTHALAMO-HYPOPHYSEAL AXIS

The hypothalamo-hypophyseal axis describes the relationship between the hypothalamus and the pituitary gland.

Hypothalamus

The hypothalamus lies below the thalamus (hence *hypo* thalamus) at the base of the brain (Fig. 9.2).

■ The main action of the hypothalamus is to control the amount and type of gonadotropic hormones secreted by the pituitary gland.

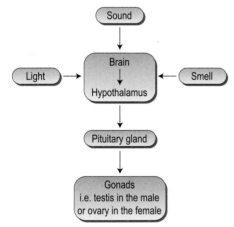

Figure 9.1 Diagram of the pathway for control of reproduction.

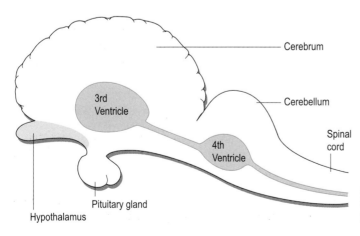

Figure 9.2 Diagram of a longitudinal section of the brain to demonstrate the position of the hypothalamus.

- It is responsible for the timing and onset of puberty.
- Sexual interest and the mating drive also depend upon neural inputs from the hypothalamus.
- It suppresses (or downgrades) the production of prolactin.

The hypothalamus receives neural input from other parts of the brain and its secretion is influenced by:

- *Daylight length.* Day length influences the pineal gland, which secretes melatonin during the hours of darkness. Melatonin is important for those species that are seasonal breeders, e.g. cats and horses.
- *Smell.* An animal's smells (pheromones) can trigger hypothalamic secretion. For example, when anoestrus sheep which are nearing the onset of their breeding season are presented to a ram the pheromones of the ram will trigger the ewe's hypothalamus to stimulate her pituitary gland to produce secretions – which result in the ewe coming into season ready to be served. This is called the 'ram effect'.
- *Nutrition.* Very thin females stop their reproductive cycles.
- *Sound.* Calling cats will bring a tom cat from some distance and trigger hypothalamic secretion, with resultant increase in the tom's libido.
- *Fear.* A male may be put off from working in the presence of another, dominant male.

The hypothalamus secretes *gonadotropin releasing hormone* (GnRH), which acts upon the pituitary gland (Box 9.1).

Pituitary gland (hypophyseal gland)

The pituitary gland is also known as the hypophyseal gland. It is an extension of the brain and has a hollow stalk that is part of the third ventricle of the brain. It can be divided into two parts:

- the anterior pituitary or anterior lobe (also called the adenohypophysis) (Box 9.2)
- the posterior pituitary or posterior lobe (also called the neurohypophysis).

Box 9.1 Secretion of gonadotropin releasing hormone (GnRH)

Gonadotropin releasing hormone is produced by the hyopothalamus. The secretions are synthesised in the neurones of the hypothalamus, transported via axonal processes and released into the blood via capillaries. Many capillary blood vessels run from the hypothalamus to the pituitary gland and join portal vessels, which end as capillaries in the pituitary gland. This blood system is called the *hypothalamic-hypophyseal portal system*.

Box 9.2 Structure of the anterior pituitary

The anterior pituitary is divided into three sections:
- pars distalis
- pars tuberalis
- pars intermedia.

The pars distalis of the anterior pituitary secretes the pituitary hormones.

Box 9.3 Non-reproductive secretions of the anterior pituitary

As well as hormones involved in reproduction the anterior pituitary secretes a number of other hormones. These are:
- somatotropin (STH), also known as growth hormone (GH) – increases tissue bulk
- thyrotropic hormone (TTH), also known as thyroid stimulating hormone (TSH) – increases secretion from the thyroid gland
- melanocyte-stimulating hormone (MSH) regulates pigmentation in amphibians and reptiles but its function in mammals is less clear

Anterior pituitary

There are four hormones secreted by the anterior pituitary which are important in the reproductive process (Box 9.3):

- luteinising hormone (LH) – also called interstitial cell stimulating hormone (ICSH)

- follicle stimulating hormone (FSH)
  (LH and FSH are called the pituitary *gonadotropins* because they act upon the gonads.)
- prolactin – also called lactogenic hormone (LTH)
- adrenocorticotropic hormone (ACTH) – stimulates the adrenal gland.

Luteinising hormone

The release of LH is stimulated by gonadotropin releasing hormone (GnRH) from the hypothalamus.
Luteinising hormone in the *female* (Box 9.4):

- high levels – a surge of LH stimulates ovulation
- low levels – assists FSH in stimulating the development of the follicle in the ovary
- low levels – supports the corpus luteum in the ovary and stimulates the production of progesterone by the luteal cells.

Luteinising hormone in the *male* (Box 9.5):

- stimulates the Leydig cells (also called interstitial cells) of the testis to secrete testosterone
- at high levels, LH acts as a *negative feedback* on the hypothalamus and reduces the amount of GnRH produced.

Follicle stimulating hormone

The release of FSH is stimulated by gonadotropin releasing hormone (GnRH) from the hypothalamus.

Follicle stimulating hormone in the *female*:

- stimulates the production of follicles in the ovary
- at high levels, FSH acts as a *negative feedback* on the hypothalamus and reduces the amount of GnRH produced.

Follicle stimulating hormone in the *male*:

- stimulates the Sertoli cells of the testis to produce androgen binding protein, which then stimulates spermatogenesis
- at high levels, FSH acts as a *negative feedback* on the hypothalamus and reduces the amount of GnRH produced.

Prolactin

The role of prolactin:

- at high levels stimulates the production of milk (Boxes 9.6, 9.7)
- at low levels maintains the corpus luteum in the ovary.

Adrenocorticotropic hormone

This hormone stimulates the adrenal cortex to release corticosteroids. Corticosteroids have a number of actions but the one we are most concerned with in reproduction is its involvement with the initiation of the cascade of events that result in parturition. The detailed physiology of parturition is dealt with below.

Posterior pituitary

The reproductive hormone produced by the posterior pituitary is oxytocin (Box 9.8). The action of oxytocin is to:

- cause milk letdown
- cause smooth muscle contraction, particularly the smooth muscle of the uterus
- act as a prostaglandin precursor, the secretion of which causes corpus luteum regression.

Box 9.4 Luteinising hormone in the female

Theca cells in the ovary respond to LH stimulation by the secretion of *testosterone*. The testosterone is converted into *oestrogen* by adjacent granulosa cells around the growing follicle. Thus as follicles grow there is an increase in oestrogen. Oestrogen is the female sex hormone. Ovulation of mature follicles in the ovary is induced by a large burst of LH secretion known as the *preovulatory LH surge*. After ovulation, cells within ovulated follicles proliferate to form *corpora lutea* (corpora lutea is the plural of corpus luteum). The cells of the corpus luteum are called *luteal cells* and these secrete *progesterone*. Progesterone is necessary for maintenance of pregnancy and LH is required for continued development and function of corpora lutea.

Box 9.5 Luteinising hormone in the male

In the testes, LH binds to receptors on Leydig cells, stimulating synthesis and secretion of *testosterone*.

Box 9.6 The control of prolactin

Secretions from the hypothalamus act to dampen or suppress the normal level of prolactin release i.e. there is a hypothalamic 'brake'. The major form of prolactin inhibition is caused by *dopamine*. Dopamine is secreted into portal blood by hypothalamic neurons. It binds to receptors on the lactotrophs (the cells that secrete prolactin) and inhibits both the synthesis and secretion of prolactin. Prolactin release is stimulated by suckling. This rise is probably due to the secretion of prolactin-releasing substances from the hypothalamus rather than a decrease in dopamine. Oestrogens provide a positive control over prolactin synthesis and secretion. The increasing blood concentrations of oestrogen during late pregnancy appear responsible for the elevated levels of prolactin that are necessary to prepare the mammary gland for lactation at the end of gestation.

Box 9.7 Action of prolactin

Prolactin induces lobulo-alveolar growth of the mammary gland. Alveoli are the clusters of cells in the mammary gland that actually secrete milk. Prolactin stimulates milk production (lactogenesis) after giving birth. Prolactin, along with cortisol and insulin, acts to stimulate transcription of the genes that encode milk proteins.

Box 9.8 Structure of the posterior pituitary and the non-reproductive hormones

The posterior pituitary (also known as the pars nervosa) consists of specialised nerve cells that secrete their hormones into the blood stream. As well as oxytocin the posterior pituitary secretes:
■ Antidiuretic hormone (ADH) – increases water reabsorption by the kidneys.

THE GONADS

The ovaries and testes are sources of reproductive hormones. These hormones are controlled by the secretions from the pituitary gland.

Testis

Two different cell types in the testis produce hormones. One cell type is Sertoli cells, which are found within the seminiferous tubules next to the spermatogonia that divide to produce sperm. The second cell type is Leydig cells. These are found between the seminiferous tubules and hence are also called interstitial cells.

Sertoli cells

The Sertoli cells of the testis are stimulated by FSH from the anterior pituitary and produce:

■ *Androgen binding protein*. This binds testosterone and thus stimulates spermatogenesis.
■ *Inhibin*. This depresses secretion of FSH by the anterior pituitary (but has no effect on LH). Thus as inhibin goes up FSH goes down. As FSH goes down inhibin goes down so that more FSH can be produced. This is an example of the 'seesaw' method of control of hormone secretion.
■ *Oestrogen*. The oestrogen is produced by converting testosterone to oestrogen. Normally there are only low levels of oestrogen produced in the male. High levels of oestrogen inhibit secretions from the anterior pituitary.

Leydig cells

The Leydig cells (also called interstitial cells) are stimulated by LH from the anterior pituitary and secrete *testosterone*. The action of testosterone is to:

■ inhibit the secretion of LH and FSH, acting as a *negative feedback*
■ stimulate the growth and activity of the male reproductive tubular genitalia (i.e. epididymis, vas deferens, ampullae, seminal vesicles, prostate, urethra, prepuce, penis) and accessory sex glands and scrotum
■ stimulate spermatogenesis in the presence of androgen binding protein

- stimulate hypertrophy of cells and organs in general; this is anabolic (i.e. building) activity
- stimulate male behaviour.

Ovary

There are a number of structures in the ovary that develop at different times during the reproductive cycle; each produces different hormones.

Granulosa cells

Granulosa cells line the tertiary or Graafian follicles in the ovary and are stimulated by FSH to produce *oestrogen*. The action of oestrogen is to:

- develop and maintain cyclic changes in the female tubular genitalia (Fallopian tube, uterine horn, uterine body, cervix and vagina)
- develop the secretory ducts of the mammary gland and uterine glands
- stimulate female oestrous behaviour (mating behaviour).

Luteal cells

The luteal cells of the corpus luteum produce

- progesterone
- relaxin
- oxytocin.

Progesterone

Known as 'the hormone of pregnancy', the action of progesterone is to:

- cause development of uterine glands in an oestrogen primed uterus
- block normal myometrial contractivity of the uterus
- stimulate glandular development of the mammary gland
- inhibit GnRH release.

The corpus luteum and secretion of progesterone is supported by LH secretion – hence LH is said to be *luteotropic*.

Relaxin

Relaxin is a hormone of pregnancy and its action is to:

- cause relaxation of the pelvic ligaments and the cervix, thus enlarging the birth canal in preparation for parturition
- suppress lactation.

Oxytocin

Although the major source of oxytocin is the posterior pituitary, luteal cells in the corpus luteum also produce small amounts of oxytocin. The action of oxytocin from luteal tissue is:

- to attach to receptors in the uterus and act as a precursor to prostaglandin, which causes regression of the corpus luteum.

Oestrogen, progesterone and testosterone are the *steroid hormones* (Figs 9.3, 9.4)

PINEAL GLAND

The pineal gland (also called the epiphysis cerebri) is attached to the roof of the third ventricle of the brain by a short stalk. It receives messages about daylight length from other parts of the brain and secretes a number of hormones, of which the most reproductively important is *melatonin*. In animals that are seasonal breeders, e.g. cats and horses, this is the hormone that 'turns on and off' the hypothalamus. Melatonin is synthesised only during the hours of darkness and its action is to suppress GnRH. The absence of GnRH means there is no stimulation of the anterior pituitary gland and so reproductive activity stops.

PHYSIOLOGY OF PARTURITION

The onset of normal parturition requires a live fetus. Secretions from the fetus trigger a cascade of events leading to parturition. The details of these events differ slightly in each species but the principles are the same:

1. The trigger for parturition is the secretion of *adrenocorticotropic hormone* from the anterior pituitary of the fetus. This secretion is brought about because of stress induced by lack of nutrients from the placenta. The fetus eventually

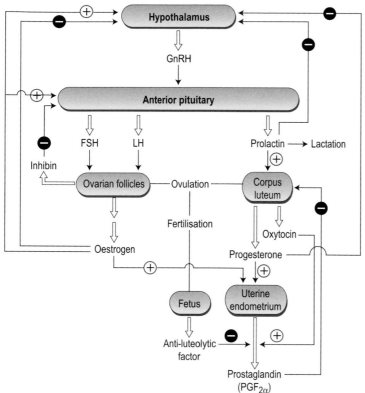

Figure 9.3 Endocrine control of female reproduction. White arrows indicate the hormone secreted. Black arrows indicate the site of the hormone action. +ve indicates stimulation. −ve indicates suppression.

reaches a size at which the placenta can no longer supply nutrients for further growth.

2. The adrenocorticotropic hormone causes the fetal and maternal adrenal cortices to release *cortisol*.

3. The raised cortisol levels stimulate the production of two enzymes, *17α hydroxylase* and *C17-20 lyase*, which, together with a third enzyme, *aromatase*, allow the conversion of progesterone to oestrogen. Aromatase is always present in the placenta but the other two enzymes are only present after stimulation by cortisol (Fig. 9.5).

4. The fall in progesterone removes the block on the contraction of the smooth muscles of the uterus (myometrium) so that the frequency and amplitude of uterine contractions increase.

5. The raised levels of oestrogen:
   - stimulate the production of oxytocin receptors in the wall of the uterus and hence the production of *prostaglandin $F_{2\alpha}$* (PGF$_{2\alpha}$),

which is luteolytic (i.e. causes regression of the corpus luteum). The presence of oxytocin receptors also allows an increase in uterine contractility.
   - cause some *relaxation of the cervix*.

6. The regression of the corpus luteum means that the progesterone levels fall even further.

7. The increased uterine contractions cause the fetus to move towards the cervix, which causes further cervical dilation.

8. Dilation of the cervix by the fetus causes release of *oxytocin* from the maternal posterior pituitary. This is called the *Ferguson's reflex*.

9. Oxytocin induces more uterine contractions, which further engage the fetus in the cervix and pelvis.

10. *Relaxin* is produced by the placenta and/or the maternal corpus luteum and causes *relaxation of the cervix*.

11. The presence of the fetus in the pelvis stimulates contraction of abdominal muscles

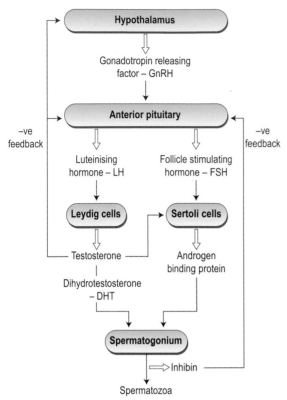

Figure 9.4 Endocrine control of male reproduction. White arrows indicate the hormone secreted. Black arrows indicate the site of the hormone action. –ve indicates that there is a suppressive effect.

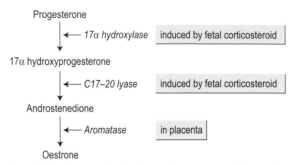

Figure 9.5 Diagram indicating the enzyme pathway for the conversion of progesterone to oestrogen at the onset of parturition.

and straining. It is the abdominal straining which is responsible for the final expulsion of the fetus through the birth canal i.e. cervix, vagina and vulva.

Parturition is usually described as having three stages (although these blend one into another):

- *First stage labour* begins with the onset of increased uterine contractions and encompasses stages 1–7 above.
- *Second stage labour* begins when the fetus enters the birth canal and abdominal straining starts. This is stage 8 above. It is the period when the fetus is expelled.
- *Third stage labour* is the expulsion of the placenta (fetal membranes) and occurs after the expulsion of the fetus in animals that have only one fetus,

or interspersed with the fetuses in litter-bearing animals.

The three stages of parturition are described in more detail for the different species in chapters 10, 11 and 12.

Terminology of parturition – presentation, position and posture

- Presentation – describes the relationship of the head and body of the fetus to the long axis of the dam. Presentation can be anterior, posterior or transverse. In anterior presentation the fetal head is coming first, posterior presentation is when the tail comes first and transverse presentation is when the fetus is across the birth canal.
- Position – describes where the fetal vertebral column is relative to the birth canal. Thus dorsal position is when the fetal spine is dorsal, ventral position is when the fetus is on its back on the floor of the pelvis.
- Posture – describes the arrangement of the fetal head and limbs.

Normal parturition is anterior presentation and dorsal position with one foreleg slightly in front of the other so that the head and two forelegs form a cone. In this presentation and posture the fetus forms a wedge, which facilitates dilation of the birth canal. It also allows compression and springing of the rib cage so that the fetus can be more easily expelled.

Lactation

The mammary glands are modified sweat glands that lie along the 'mammary ridge' either side of the midline of the ventral abdomen. The number of glands that develop depends on the species.

Cats and dogs have five pairs of glands along the ventral midline; the mare has one pair of glands between the hind legs. Each gland has a teat and the teats have a different number of canals depending upon the species. The bitch and queen have 5/6 ducts per teat; the mare has 2/3 ducts per teat.

Development of the mammary glands is triggered by rising levels of prolactin and milk letdown is triggered by oxytocin. The milk released in the first few hours after parturition is called colostrum. Colostrum has a high level of antibodies, which are transferred to the offspring when they suckle. Colostrum therefore conveys passive immunity to the newborn, depending upon what immunity has been developed by the dam. The antibodies are absorbed undamaged by the newborn in the first few hours of life because the pH of their stomach is neutral. As soon as the stomach pH drops the antibodies are destroyed and the newborn receives no more passive immunity. It is therefore very important for the newborn to receive as much colostrum as possible as soon as possible after birth.

10

Reproductive physiology of the dog

Core information: **The bitch is monoestrus. There is a prolonged pro-oestrus when follicles are growing and the dominant hormone is oestrogen. The follicles begin to luteinise and secrete progesterone before ovulation. During oestrus, when the female will accept the male, the dominant hormone is progesterone. The oocyte takes about 48 hours after ovulation before it is mature and ready for fertilisation. The life of the corpus luteum is shorter during pregnancy than non-pregnancy. The dominant hormone during pregnancy is progesterone. The precipitous decline in progesterone at parturition stimulates prolactin release and lactation.**

THE BITCH

Reproduction in the bitch is not governed by day length and thus it cannot be said to be seasonal.

Puberty is defined as when the bitch shows the first oestrus. It occurs from 5 to 18 months old, depending upon breed and sire (i.e. genetics), and nutrition. Smaller breeds tend to have an earlier puberty than the larger breeds. Bitches come into oestrus and then go out again and so bitches are said to be *monoestrus*. There is quite a variation between bitches in the interoestrous interval, although most bitches establish their own rhythm. As the bitch ages the interoestrous interval becomes more irregular.

Most bitches have two reproductively active periods a year (their 'season') but this does depend on the breed. For example the Basenji has only one season a year, Collies have a season approximately every 9 months and German Shepherds about every 26 weeks. A bitch's 'season' consists of two physiologically different periods (pro-oestrus and true oestrus) whist the annual cycle consists of four periods (pro-oestrus, true oestrus, metoestrus and anoestrus).

The 'season' begins with a period of follicular growth, called *pro-oestrus*. This lasts for 7–9 days but the length can be very variable both within and between individual bitches. During this time the bitch is attractive to the male and he may attempt to mount and serve her but she will not allow mating. The predominant hormone at this stage is *oestrogen* (Box 10.1). The raised levels of oestrogen cause:

- production of pheromones that make the bitch attractive to the male
- development of numerous capillaries in the uterus and blood seepage into the uterine lumen (this blood is discharged via the vagina and is what breeders mean when they say that the bitch is 'blood spotting'; technically the bitch can be said to have a *serosanguinous vaginal discharge*)
- oedematous swelling of the vulval lips and perineal region so that the vulva is enlarged and protrudes
- oedematous swelling of the wall of the vagina so that the lining of the vagina becomes swollen and glistening
- increase in the number of layers of cells of the epithelial lining of the vagina (after prolonged oestrogen exposure the outer vaginal cell layers die, become cornified and slough off into the vaginal lumen)
- a negative feedback on the hypothalamus and pituitary gland to stop further FSH.

As the follicles mature, pro-oestrus develops into *true oestrus* and the bitch begins to allow the dog to mount. True oestrus can be of very variable length but averages about 7–9 days. This is when the bitch will accept the dog's advances and allow mating. The peak oestrogen levels trigger more LH secretion by the anterior pituitary (and thus at this one point oestrogen has a positive feedback on the anterior pituitary). The follicles mature and begin to luteinise prior to ovulation (i.e. there is preovulatory luteinisation of the follicles). At this stage oestrogen levels fall and progesterone levels rise (Box 10.2). The results of these hormone changes are:

- full cornification of the epithelial lining of the vaginal epithelium
- reduction in perineal swelling
- reduction in vaginal mucous swelling and oedema
- behavioural oestrus – the bitch plays with the dog and allows him to mount, she will move the tail to one side to facilitate intromission (this is known as 'slipping' the tail).

The high levels of oestrogen at the end of pro-oestrus stimulate LH secretion by the anterior pituitary gland. This starts the luteinisation of the follicle before ovulation. Eventually there is an LH peak, or spike, and this causes ovulation (Box 10.3).

During true oestrus the bitch solicits the male's attention and offers her rear for him to smell. She

---

Box 10.2 Progesterone in true oestrus in the bitch

The bitch is unusual in that the follicles undergo preovulatory luteinisation. Thus oestrogen levels fall and progesterone levels rise *before* ovulation. This is very unusual. In all other species progesterone levels do not rise until after ovulation. We can measure this preovulatory rise of progesterone in the bitch and predict when ovulation is about to take place. Thus it is used as a test to pinpoint the best time to serve the bitch.

Box 10.1 Production of oestrogen

During pro-oestrus the ovarian follicles begin to grow in response to stimulation by follicle stimulating hormone (FSH) from the anterior pituitary. The FSH is produced in response to gonadotropin releasing hormone (GnRH) from the hypothalamus. The granulosa cells of the developing follicles secrete oestrogen.

Box 10.3 Ovulation in the bitch

Ovulation occurs approximately 40–50 hours after the LH surge but the egg is not ready for fertilisation at this stage. It requires a further two days of maturation in the uterine tube (also called the oviduct or Fallopian tube) before the egg (oocyte) is capable of being fertilised.

will lift the tail to one side and flex the back so that the vulva is presented to the male. This behaviour is due to the decline in oestrogen and rise in progesterone.

Ovulation of a follicle results in the formation of a corpus luteum. When the follicle collapses to allow the release of the egg the leuteinising granulosa cells become the luteal cells and invade the cavity to form the corpus luteum. Luteal cells secrete progesterone.

Different breeds of dogs will ovulate different numbers of follicles – generally speaking, bigger breeds have larger litters. Each ovulated follicle forms a corpus luteum so there are a number of corpora lutea in each ovary after ovulation.

Once ovulation and fertilisation occurs the bitch stops accepting the dog and the 'season' stops. However, the bitch is still hormonally active and this stage is called *metoestrus*. This is the period of growth and dominance of the corpora lutea where the predominant hormone is *progesterone*. The action of progesterone is to:

- act as a negative feedback to inhibit FSH secretion
- cause proliferation of uterine glands and support pregnancy
- cause reduction in the number of layers of epithelial cells in the vagina
- cause reduction of cornification of vaginal epithelial cells
- stimulate an invasion of polymorphonucleocytes into the vaginal mucosa to mop up the sloughed keratinised epithelial cells.

Metoestrus lasts for a long time (70–90 days) during which there is development and then gradual decline in the corpora lutea. If the animal is served and becomes pregnant then there is an induced luteolysis 63 days after fertilisation to allow parturition (see below).

Metoestrus fades into *anoestrus*, which is the period of ovarian inactivity until the next pro-oestrus. The triggers that start pro-oestrus again are not fully understood (Fig. 10.1).

Determination of time to mate

There is a great variation in the length of the pro-oestrous period and the time at which ovulation

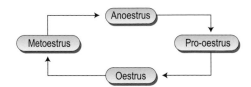

Figure 10.1 Oestrous cycle in the bitch.

occurs in true oestrus. To ensure that the bitch is served at the optimum time it is advisable that owners allow the dog to serve the bitch every other day until the bitch will not stand to be mounted. Whilst this management is likely to maximise the chances of fertilisation it is not always practical. This is because:

- it is costly if the bitch owner has to pay for each service
- it is wasteful of the dog's reproductive capacity (see below) and will reduce the number of bitches he can successfully serve.

Thus, it has become desirable to be able to establish when ovulation takes place in order to co-ordinate mating with this event.

Measurement of the LH peak in peripheral blood
Measurement of LH levels to identify the LH peak would be the best way to identify an imminent ovulation because ovulation is closely correlated with this LH surge. However, the LH surge is transitory and so multiple blood samples, perhaps as frequently as every 10–15 minutes, have to be made in order not to miss the LH peak. For practical purposes this is not a viable technique for most breeding bitches.

Character of vaginal mucosa
During pro-oestrus the vaginal mucosa is oedematous, rounded, pink and glistening. As oestrogen levels fall and progesterone levels rise the character of the vaginal mucosa changes. The mucosa becomes more shrunken and wrinkled. These changes can be viewed with a vaginoscope or an endoscope and can be used to assess the hormonal status of the animal. However the changes are not sufficiently precise to predict accurately the LH surge and ovulation and therefore, although

helpful in establishing the optimum time to mate, such changes alone are not sufficient.

Vaginal epithelial cytology

This used to be the commonest method of predicting ovulation. The rapid changes in the type of dominant hormone during the reproductive cycle of the bitch cause changes in the vaginal epithelium, which can be monitored by means of vaginal cytology. During pro-oestrus the predominant cell type is red blood cells and the epithelial cells are rounded with clear nuclei (Fig. 10.2). As the oestrogen levels rise the number of layers of epithelial cells lining the vagina increase and begin to keratinise. A vaginal smear at the optimum time for service will show more than 80% of darkly staining, angular anuclear epithelial cells with few, if any, red blood cells (Fig. 10.3).

When oestrus is over, sloughed cells are removed by an invasion of polymorphonucleocytes (PMNs) and so the predominant cell type in metoestrus is PMNs (Fig. 10.4). The test is simple and minimally invasive. This examination is quite good at defining the optimum time to mate. However, vaginal mucosa growth and keratinisation follows the pro-oestral rise in oestrogen by about 3–4 days and is completed in 5–10 days. Thus peak keratinisation may not always correlate with the LH peak and ovulation and so once again this test is not 100% accurate (Box 10.4, Table 10.1).

Measurement of peripheral blood progesterone

This is currently the most accurate method of predicting ovulation. The bitch is unusual in that progesterone levels begin to rise *before* ovulation takes place. Therefore it is possible to measure the rise in progesterone and predict when ovulation is about to take place. There is a qualitative Elisa kit for the measurement of blood progesterone (Ovucheck PreMate®) that can be used in the practice. Alternatively, a number of laboratories offer a quantitative assay. Once the progesterone levels reach 7.5ng/ml ovulation is imminent. Sometimes anovulatory cycles occur, in which case

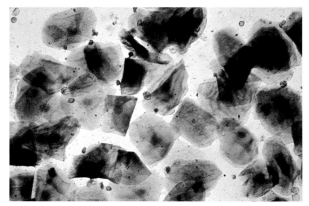

Figure 10.3 Vaginal smear from a bitch in oestrus showing angular, anuclear darkly-staining keratinised cells.

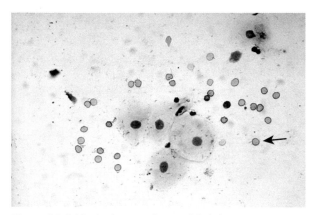

Figure 10.2 Vaginal smear from a bitch in pro-oestrus showing the red blood cells (arrowed) and nucleated epithelial cells.

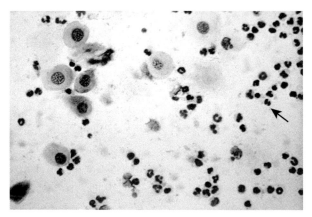

Figure 10.4 Vaginal smear from a bitch in metoestrus showing polymorphonucleocytes (arrowed) (the characteristic cell type at this stage) and nucleated epithelial cells.

progesterone levels fail to continue to rise above about 7.5ng/ml and just decline over the next few days. It is therefore advisable to measure progesterone levels again once the bitch has gone out of oestrus to check that ovulation has taken place.

Pregnancy

Fertilisation takes place in the uterine tube and the early embryo is in the uterine horn by 9–10 days later. Implantation occurs at about 19–20 days post-fertilisation.

Progesterone is the dominant hormone of pregnancy but there is little or no difference in the hormonal levels in pregnant and non-pregnant bitches. Therefore, all bitches have a kind of pseudopregnancy after each season. (This may be why some breeders think that their bitches are pregnant when they are not. They see the same changes in behaviour and body mass early on, influenced by the raised progesterone levels.)

Relaxin is a pregnancy specific hormone produced by the ovary and the placenta. It rises gradually in the last two-thirds of pregnancy and is detectable from about day 25 of gestation.

The *gestation length* is 63(±1) days relative to the time of fertilisation but can be very variable (56–72 days) relative to the time of *service* because of the variation between the time of service and fertilisation. This often causes confusion and/or problems for breeders and veterinary surgeons because it can be difficult to know when to intervene to deliver puppies if there are problems at parturition.

Pregnancy diagnosis
There are a number of ways in which a pregnancy can be detected:

- abdominal palpation
- transabdominal ultrasonography
- transabdominal radiography
- peripheral blood relaxin levels
- Doppler ultrasound
- transabdominal auscultation.

Abdominal palpation
At about 3–4 weeks the individual fetal swellings can be palpated through the abdominal wall as discrete 'bumps', 12–15mm in diameter, along the uterine horn. Ease of detection depends upon how relaxed the bitch is during the procedure, how fat she is and how many puppies are present. Single pups can easily be missed. At 5–6 weeks after conception the swellings coalesce and it is difficult to palpate pregnancy accurately. After 6–7 weeks the fetuses can again be palpated because

---

Box 10.4 Collection of a vaginal epithelial cells

- A sterile swab is inserted into the anterior vagina, via a sterile guide. Some clinicians prefer a dry swab, others a damp swab.
- The swab is rotated against the wall of the anterior vagina in order to collect plenty of cells.
- The swab is withdrawn and dabbed onto a microscope slide in order to transfer vaginal cells. It is better not to roll the swab because this tends to tear the cells.
- The preparation is allowed to dry and then fixed and stained.
- A commonly available stain in the practice environment is Diff-Quik®.

Table 10.1 Changes in vaginal cytology during oestrus in the bitch

	Red blood cells	Squamous epithelial cells	Cornified epithelial cells	Polymorphonucleocytes
Pro-oestrus	+++	+++	–	–
Oestrus	(+)	+	+++	–
Metoestrus	–	++	–	+++
Anoestrus	–	+	–	–

Key: - cell type absent, (+) cell type may be present, + scant number of cells, ++ moderate number of cells, +++ the major cell type present.

ossification has taken place and fetal heads can be identified. At this stage it is difficult to determine the number of puppies.

Transabdominal ultrasonography

From 3 weeks onwards fetal fluids and fetuses can be detected by real time transabdominal ultrasound. A similar technique is used in human pregnancy diagnosis. The technique has the big advantage of being able to determine fetal heart beat and hence the viability of the fetus. Transabdominal ultrasonography is currently the most reliable method of pregnancy diagnosis.

Transabdominal radiography

After 6–7 weeks radiography can be used to determine fetal skeletons. Fetal viability is more difficult to confirm because fetal heart beat cannot be detected. However, if there has been fetal death and autolysis has begun then skeletal degeneration and putrefying gases can be detected.

Peripheral blood relaxin levels

Relaxin is a pregnancy-specific hormone found in the blood, which, in the bitch, begins to rise 21–26 days after conception. An Elisa assay kit, ReproCheck Relaxin®, is commercially available for use in the practice.

Doppler ultrasound

This system works by firing sound waves through the abdominal wall, these are reflected at a different frequency when they hit moving fluid such as blood in fetal umbilical veins or fetal heart. This method has now been superseded by real-time ultrasound scanning.

Transabdominal auscultation

Late on in pregnancy it is possible to hear the fetal heart beats with a stethoscope. Fetal heart rate is about twice that of the dam.

Parturition

High levels of progesterone during pregnancy dampen the normal contractions of the uterus. Parturition is instigated by luteolysis and reduction in the level of progesterone. This is triggered by signals from the fetus (see physiology of parturition). Raised levels of corticosteroids are seen one day prepartum. There are no raised oestrogen levels at parturition in the bitch and so the exact mechanism of parturition is not fully understood. There are three stages to parturition or labour.

First stage labour

This is the period of increased uterine muscle contraction. It can last for 6–36 hours but is usually approximately 12 hours long. It is usually preceded by a transient drop in deep body temperature of 2°C.

■ The bitch will appear restless and nervous. She often has a wish to make a nest and will look for quiet and familiar places. She may pant and keep looking at her flanks, which is an indication that uterine contractions are occurring.
■ The vagina relaxes and the cervix dilates.
■ The fetus rotates so that the head is pointing towards the cervix. (Not all fetuses complete this rotation. Transverse puppies can cause dystocia but posterior presentation is often not a problem because of the relative small size of the fetus and large size of the maternal pelvis.)

Second stage labour

This is the period of voluntary abdominal wall contraction and expulsion of the fetus. It is usually completed within 3–12 hours. The bitch lies on her side and there is visible abdominal straining. The first puppy should appear within 2–4 hours of the start of the abdominal straining. If there is strong abdominal straining for 20–30 minutes then a pup should appear. The interval between each puppy varies but should not be more than 2–4 hours (or 30 minutes if there has been strong abdominal straining).

There is an expulsion of greenish fluid when the abdominal straining starts. This is the allantochorionic fluid and is often referred to as 'the breaking of the water bag'. The greenish colour is the result of the pigments at the margins of the zonary placenta in the bitch (Fig. 10.5). The puppy may be expelled within the amniotic membrane but this is usually quickly broken and eaten by the bitch. The bitch will lick the puppy – this not only

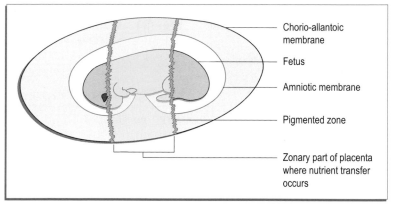

Figure 10.5 Diagrammatic representation of the arrangement of fetal membranes in the dog and cat. The amniotic membrane forms a sac, which contains amniotic fluid and surrounds the embryo. The chorio-allantoic membrane forms a second sac, which contains chorio-allantoic fluid. A central band of the chorio-allantoic membrane attaches to the uterus of the dam. This forms the zonary placenta where nutrients are transferred. At the edge of the zonary placenta is a pigmented area, which is green in the dog and red/brown in the cat.

cleans and dries the pup but also stimulates it to breathe.

Third stage labour

This is the period of expulsion of the placenta (fetal membranes). It usually occurs within 15 minutes of expulsion of the pup although it is not uncommon for two or three puppies to be born, followed by their placentae. Normally it is best to leave the parturient bitch in peace. However, if she is exhausted or a young and inexperienced bitch it may be necessary to attend to the newborn puppy (neonate) in order to ensure its survival.

Nursing assistance at parturition

- The amniotic membrane may need to be broken to allow the puppy to breathe.
- Vigorous rubbing may be necessary to dry the puppy, to warm it, and to encourage breathing.
- The fetal fluids may be blocking the airways. These should be cleared either by gentle sucking with a plastic pipette or by gently swinging the pup downwards. *This procedure must be carried out with care as it may cause brain haemorrhage.*
- The umbilical cord can be clamped with sterile forceps and cut with sterile scissors, leaving approximately 4 cm attached to the pup. If there is umbilical bleeding it may be necessary to ligate the umbilicus with absorbable material.
- Healthy puppies will find the teat and suck vigorously but some puppies need to be helped onto a teat.

Parturition is usually completed within 6 hours of the onset of second stage labour. Anything longer than 12 hours should be considered abnormal.

Prolactin levels start to rise from mid-gestation until parturition. There is a surge of prolactin during the precipitous drop in progesterone prepartum and this triggers lactation. Suckling by the puppies stimulates *oxytocin* release from the posterior pituitary gland and initiates milk letdown.

Lactation

During pregnancy the mammary glands begin to develop in response to the gradual increase in the levels of prolactin. At parturition there is a precipitous drop in progesterone and prolactin levels rise (Box 10.5). Lactation lasts for 6–9 weeks – during this period prolactin levels remain elevated. Pregnancy and lactation do not seem to increase the interval until the next oestrus.

Box 10.5 Hormones of lactation

Prolactin stimulates the synthesis of milk and oxytocin allows milk letdown. Maintenance of lactation also requires cortisol and insulin.

Box 10.6 Pseudopregnancy and pseudocyesis

Strictly speaking, *pseudopregnancy* is when the bitch has the appearance of pregnancy even although she is not. All bitches show this to some degree because under the influence of progesterone the uterus is enlarging to prepare for the fetus. In some bitches this is so pronounced that owners are convinced that the animal really is pregnant because of the increase in weight and the change in body conformation. Some bitches go even further and show signs of nest making, the mammary glands enlarge and they begin to lactate. The onset of lactation without parturition is *pseudocyesis*. However, lactation when the bitch is not pregnant is commonly referred to by owners and veterinary surgeons as pseudopregnancy.

Pseudopregnancy/pseudocyesis

It is not uncommon for some non-pregnant bitches to begin to lactate some weeks after their season. This is commonly called 'pseudopregnancy'. It is a misleading name because the bitch does not show signs of *pregnancy* but is lactating. The more correct term is *pseudocyesis* – lactation in the absence of pregnancy. It occurs in the bitch because of the normal physiology of the corpus luteum in this species. The corpus luteum in the bitch is usually active for longer when the animal is *not* pregnant than when it is (Box 10.6). In the pregnant animal the corpora lutea are actively caused to regress by a chain of events triggered by the mature fetus. This causes a precipitous decline in progesterone. In the non-pregnant animal the levels of progesterone normally decline slowly as the corpora lutea slowly degenerate.

Pseudocyesis is caused either by a more precipitous decline in progesterone at the end of the normal life of the corpus luteum or a greater sensitivity in some animals to the normal decline. The effect is to cause release of prolactin and the induction of lactation.

Manipulation of reproduction in the bitch

It is possible to manipulate reproduction by manipulating the physiology. The following procedures are commonly carried out to manipulate reproduction.

Spaying

In the UK spaying is the removal of the ovaries, uterine horns and uterine body. This is an ovariohysterectomy and results in a permanent stoppage of the reproductive cycle. To stop the cycle it is only necessary to remove the ovaries, which is commonly done in continental Europe. Removal of the ovaries alone is called an ovariectomy. Physiologically, it is the removal of the female reproductive hormone *oestrogen*, produced in the ovaries, which stops the normal cyclic events. Removal of the uterus is carried out to ensure that there is no subsequent infection of the organ.

Interruption of behavioural oestrus

If a bitch has started to develop follicles, i.e. she is in pro-oestrus, continued development of the follicles can be blocked by giving exogenous *progesterone*. Progesterone blocks the production of FSH, which is necessary for the development of follicles, so the bitch's 'season' is blocked.

Progesterone can be given to the bitch in the form of daily tablets (e.g. Ovarid®) or by injection (e.g. Delvosteron®), which lasts for a few months. When the treatment with progesterone stops, the bitch can cycle normally. The advantage of daily tablets is that the treatment can be stopped quickly. The disadvantage is that it is more trouble to ensure that the animal actually gets the medication. The advantage of the injectable progesterone is that a single injection will last for a number of months. The disadvantage is that once it has been given the dose cannot be taken away.

Postponement of oestrus

The onset of oestrus can be postponed by giving *progesterone*. The action is similar to interruption of behavioural oestrus (see above). The progesterone blocks FSH and so follicles do not develop. Progesterone can again be administered either in tablet form or by injections.

Induction of oestrus

The mechanism of induction of oestrus in the bitch is not well understood. However it can be achieved by giving *anti-prolactin* (e.g. Galastop®). Prolactin suppresses LH and FSH secretion but anoestrus bitches do not have high levels of prolactin, so the mechanism of action of exogenous anti-prolactin is not known.

Treatment of pseudocyesis (pseudopregnancy)

Lactation in the absence of a pregnancy can be suppressed by treatment with *progesterone*, which blocks the secretion of prolactin, or by the administration of a specific *anti-prolactin* (e.g. Galastop®). The latter is the treatment of choice.

Termination of pregnancy

A pregnancy can be terminated in a number of ways, e.g.

- administration of a specific *anti-progestogen* (e.g. Alazin®) – progesterone is necessary to support pregnancy
- removal of the corpora lutea which produce progesterone, e.g. by using *anti-prolactin* (e.g. Galastop®) since prolactin is necessary to support the corpus luteum
- a combination of *anti-progestogen* and *anti-prolactin*.

Induction of parturition

Parturition can be induced by administering *corticosteroids*; these stimulate the production of enzymes that convert progesterone to oestrogen. This increases uterine contractions and triggers the cascade of events that lead to parturition. This technique is only effective if there are viable placentae and the uterine myometrium is capable of contracting. It is therefore not suitable for cases of uterine inertia. Furthermore, live-born puppies will only be produced if the induction is carried out close to term.

Induction of milk let down

If there has been mammary development but the milk is not being secreted this can be induced by administering *oxytocin*.

All of the above manipulations can have undesirable side effects and such manipulations should only be carried out by a veterinary surgeon.

THE DOG

Male dogs are sexually active throughout the year without any influence of season.

Puberty is defined as when the dog releases spermatozoa in the ejaculate. It occurs at between 9–12 months old but sexual maturity is not reached until about 15–16 months.

Normal testes

The testes descend into the scrotum a few days after birth but may be difficult to palpate at this time because they can easily be withdrawn back into the inguinal ring. They are normally permanently within the scrotum by 8 weeks of age but testis descent can be delayed until as late as 6–8 months. After this age, if a testis has not descended it will not do so.

Spermatozoal output is related to testis size and this is related to body size. Thus large dogs have larger testes and produce more spermatozoa than small dogs.

Spermatogenesis

In the male fetus primordial germ cells divide mitotically to increase in number. During the pre-pubertal period these differentiate into spermatogonia. There is then no further development until puberty.

Spermiocytogenesis is the first stage of spermatogenesis:

- Spermatogonia on the basement membrane of the seminiferous tubules divide mitotically. This produces new spermatogonia and primary spermatocytes.
- The primary spermatocytes undergo meiotic division to produce secondary spermatocytes.

- The secondary spermatocytes divide meiotically to produce spherical spermatids.

Spermiogenesis is the second stage of spermatogenesis:

- The spherical spermatids mature into elongated spermatids.

Spermiation is the final stage of spermatogenesis and is the process of release of the elongated spermatids into the lumen of the seminiferous tubules as spermatozoa. The average time required for spermatogenesis in the dog is 62 days (see Fig. 1.16).

Cryptorchidism and cryptorchids

Failure of the testes to descend into the scrotum is called *cryptorchidism* and the animal is said to be a cryptorchid (Box 10.7). Failure of only one testis to descend is *unilateral* cryptorchidism. Unilateral cryptorchids can be fertile because the descended testis will produce spermatozoa (Box 10.8).

There is more than one reason for cryptorchidism but it can be a genetically influenced condition. In some cases it is said to be due to sex-limited autosomal genes but it may also be polygenic. Boxers, Bulldogs, Chihuahuas, Miniature Dachshunds, Old English Sheepdogs, Pekingese, Pomeranian, Toy and Miniature Poodles, Miniature Schnauzers, Shetland Sheepdogs and Yorkshire Terriers are breeds believed to be at increased risk of cryptorchidism.

It is recommended that unilateral cryptorchids are not used as stud dogs. Furthermore their littermates, including the females, are also at risk of passing on some of the genes involved in cryptorchidism and so it is advisable not to breed from these animals either.

Accessory glands of the dog

The *prostate* is the only accessory gland in the dog. It is located caudal to the neck of the bladder and encircles the urethra. The prostate is androgen dependent – its size increases with testosterone secretion and decreases when there are raised levels of oestrogen. As the animal ages the size of the

> ### Box 10.7 Cryptorchidism and spermatogenesis
>
> Testes that remain in the abdomen do not produce spermatozoa because spermatogenesis is temperature dependent and can only take place below the normal deep body temperature. Testes in the scrotum are at a lower temperature and so spermatogenesis can take place.

> ### Box 10.8 Cryptorchid testes and tumours
>
> Testes that are retained in the abdomen are at normal body temperature – which is higher than optimum for these organs. This is believed to be the reason why abdominal testes are more likely to develop tumours. Tumour development in retained testes is more of a problem in the dog than in the tom cat.

prostate increases – older dogs often show clinical signs of *benign prostatic hyperplasia*. The clinical signs are those related to the increased size of the organ and can include constipation and/or straining on defaecation.

Mating

The technical term for mating is coitus. In the dog it is a protracted procedure and can last up to 20 minutes:

- The dog first mounts the bitch from the rear and grabs the pelvic bones with his front paws.
- He starts to make exploratory thrusting movements with the penis, seeking the vulval lips. During this time the penis is partially erect – this is when intromission occurs.
- Full erection is achieved within the vagina with elongation of the penis and enlargement of the bulbus glandis. The penis is then 'locked' in the bitch's vagina by contraction of the vaginal sphincter behind the swollen bulbus glandis of the penis. When the penis is fully erect the sperm-rich fraction of the ejaculate is produced (see below). Thrusting usually stops when ejaculation is taking place.

- After the sperm-rich fraction the dog usually turns and dismounts to face backwards, whilst retaining the penis in the vagina. This is the 'tie.' It is not necessary for the dog to turn or to achieve a tie in order to have a complete ejaculation and normal mating. Some dogs prefer not to turn and remain on the bitch. If the dog is heavy this can become uncomfortable for the bitch.
- For the 'tie' to be broken the vaginal sphincter must relax and the bulbus glandis swelling must reduce. Forced separation of the dog and bitch before penile swelling has reduced can cause damage and pain to one or both animals.

The *ejaculate* can be divided into three fractions (Box 10.9):

- The *presperm fraction* (1st fraction) consists of clear fluid with little or no spermatozoa. The volume can vary from just a few drops to as much as 10 ml. It is produced whilst the dog is thrusting and attempting intromission.
- The *sperm rich fraction* (2nd fraction) is milky in colour due to the presence of numerous spermatozoa. The volume can vary and range from 1ml to 2ml.

Box 10.9 Normal ejaculate characteristics of the dog

- Volume:
  - 1st fraction: 1–10ml
  - 2nd fraction: 1–2ml
  - 3rd fraction: 1–20ml*
- % motile sperm: >70%
- % morphologically normal sperm: >80%
- Number of sperm per ejaculate: $>200 \times 10^6$

*The volume of the third fraction is intrinsically variable but will also depend on how much is actually collected by the operator.

- The third fraction is *prostatic fluid*. This is clear fluid with few spermatozoa. Prostatic fluid is produced in a pulsatile manner and can be secreted for 15 minutes or more.

Manipulation of reproduction in the dog

It is more difficult to manipulate male reproduction than female reproduction.

Surgical castration

Castration is the removal of the testes. Apart from removing the source of sperm production, the physiological result is also to remove the source of testosterone. Thus the effect is seen on the testosterone dependent accessory glands. In the dog this is the prostate gland, which becomes smaller after castration. Removal of testosterone also reduces the amount of tissue build-up, particularly muscle, since testosterone is an anabolic steroid.

Chemical castration

This term is used to describe the blocking of testosterone action without actually removing the testes. Although the source of spermatozoa is not removed the production of spermatozoa is stopped because testosterone is needed to permit the production of sperm. The effects of testosterone can be blocked by *oestrogen* or *progestogens* (Box 10.10). A common progestogen used to suppress sexual activity in the dog is Tardak®.

Box 10.10 Progestogens

A progestogen is a substance that has progesterone-like activity. Therefore, progesterone is a progestogen but other progestogens are not progesterone.

11
Reproductive physiology of the cat

Chapter contents

Core information: **The cat is seasonally polyoestrus with oestrous cycles stimulated by increase in day length. Ovulation is induced by mating. An infertile mating will produce a pseudopregnancy.**

THE QUEEN

The female cat (queen) is seasonally polyoestrous. She starts to cycle with increase in daylight length. This is controlled by *melatonin* secretion from the pineal gland. If queens are kept in a steady 16 hours of daylight, as is often the case in breeding establishments, they will cycle throughout the year.

The queen differs from the bitch in that she is an induced ovulator. That is, ovulation is triggered by the act of mating (coitus). In the absence of mating the mature follicle regresses without ovulating (this is also a characteristic of the female ferret and rabbit).

Puberty

The age of onset of puberty varies and can range from 4 to 18 months. The commonest age when queens start to cycle is 6–9 months. The variation depends upon:

- body weight – most cats start to cycle when they are 2.3–2.5kg in weight.
- the time of year of birth – queens are more likely to come into season when there is increasing daylight length. If a female reaches the right body weight in autumn or winter she often does not come into season until the following spring when the daylight length begins to increase.

■ Breed – oriental short-haired breeds such as Siamese and Burmese tend to start puberty at a lower body weight than long haired-breeds such as Persians. Therefore the background genetics of the animal is playing a role here.

The oestrous cycle

In the absence of mating and ovulation the oestrous cycle can be divided into pro-oestrus, oestrus, interoestrus and anoestrus.

■ *Pro-oestrus* is difficult to detect. Therefore pro-oestrus and oestrus are often taken together and just called oestrus. Pro-oestrus is often considered to be the first few days of heat (1–4 days) when the queen is calling but will not accept the male's advances (Box 11.1). During this time the ovarian follicles are beginning to grow but oestrogen levels are still fairly low.
■ *Oestrus* is the period (3–7days) when the female will accept the male (tom). It is the period when the follicles are mature and there is a maximum level of secretion of *oestrogens* from the follicles. The raised levels of oestrogen are necessary to:
  – induce oestrous behaviour
  – prime the anterior pituitary for the luteinising hormone (LH) surge that causes ovulation.

In the absence of mating the follicles regress, oestrogen levels fall, oestrus suddenly ceases and the queen will stop calling.

■ *Interoestrus* is the period between one oestrus and the next. In this stage the oestrogen levels are basal. In the absence of mating and ovulation the queen will come back into season every 10–14 days. (Thus, the oestrous cycle is approximately 21 days i.e. about 7 days of pro-oestrus and oestrus plus 14 days of interoestrus.)
■ *Anoestrus* is the period during the winter when there is no ovarian activity. This quiescent time is due to the secretion of *melatonin* from the pineal gland. Melatonin is secreted during the hours of darkness and suppresses the release of gonadotropin releasing hormone (GnRH) from the hypothalamus. Thus the anterior pituitary gland does not release the gonadotropins [follicle stimulating hormone (FSH), and LH] that would stimulate the ovaries.

Mating

When the queen is in pro-oestrus/early oestrus she attracts the male with her vocalisation and oestrous odour but does not allow mating. During this time several toms may gather around the female until she is receptive. When the female is eventually receptive she will allow several matings in quick succession, not always from the same male.

The tom will grab the queen by the scruff of the neck with his teeth and mount whilst she paddles and presents the vulva. Intromission and ejaculation is swift and the female emits a characteristic yowl when the male dismounts. This expression of pain is believed to be caused by stimulation of the vagina by the penile spines. The queen shows what is called the 'rage reaction' i.e. she takes a swipe at the tom with her front paw and rolls on her back and licks the vulva. Experienced toms quickly retreat to a safe distance after dismounting but inexperienced toms can be injured by an aggressive female.

Ovulation

The successive matings are important to trigger ovulation and so remounting can be allowed after as little as 10 minutes. Vaginal stimulation at mating causes a reflex release of GnRH from the hypothalamus, which triggers *luteinising hormone*

Box 11.1 Calling in cats

Calling is the term used to describe the vocalisation of the queen when she is in heat, together with the particular behaviour with which she will solicit the tom's attention. She will rub against the furniture, roll on the ground and be very affectionate towards the owner. When stroked she will crouch with the fore legs, raise the hind legs, deflect the tail and present the vulva whilst paddling with all four feet. During this time she will make loud yowling meows, which attract the tom. Owners sometimes think that the animal is in pain and will seek veterinary help.

release from the anterior pituitary. LH release is primed by the raised oestrogen levels present in oestrus. Successive matings induce higher and higher peaks of LH until the ovulatory surge of LH occurs. It is important that successive matings occur in a short period of time otherwise the LH levels drop and an ovulatory peak is not achieved (Fig. 11.1). The LH surge lasts longer after multiple matings and optimum levels are obtained if there are four matings within 2–4 hours. Ovulation rate (i.e. the number of follicles ovulated) varies depending upon breed and the number and timing of matings.

After ovulation the queen goes out of oestrus in 24–48 hours and corpora lutea develop on the ovaries from each ovulated follicle.

Induction of ovulation is easier in some breeds than others. The Oriental breeds, e.g. Siamese, require fewer matings to stimulate ovulation than, for example, domestic shorthairs. On average about four matings are required to induce ovulation but some queens will ovulate after only one mating.

In some circumstances ovulation will occur without a mating taking place. Some cats can be induced to ovulate by stroking the back and tail. This is particularly true of the oriental breeds. Furthermore, cats kept in colonies may ovulate without being mated. This may be due to the pheromonal activity within the colony or the activity of other female cats.

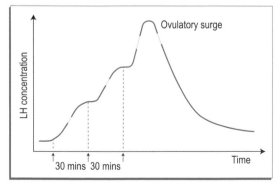

Figure 11.1 Diagrammatic representation of changes in luteinising hormone (LH) in the female cat after successive matings that result in the preovulatory surge. Arrows indicate a mating event.

Ovulation without fertilisation

After ovulation the corpora lutea form and produce *progesterone*. If mating takes place without fertilisation then the corpora will continue to develop and produce progesterone. In the cat, the life of the corpus luteum in the absence of a fetus is shorter than if there is a pregnancy. (This is different from the bitch where the corpus luteum remains for a longer period if the bitch is non-pregnant than when she is pregnant.) In the cat, in the absence of a fetus the corpora lutea continue to produce progesterone for 25 days and then regress so that progesterone levels are basal after about 30–40 days. This could be considered to be a *pseudopregnancy* but unlike the bitch it is not associated with behavioural changes such as nest making or lactation.

After regression of the corpora lutea there is a short inter-oestrus period when reproductive hormones are basal. FSH levels then begin to rise again and the queen will come back into heat if it is the breeding season. However if it is autumn and there is decreasing daylight length, the queen will go into anoestrus after regression of the corpora lutea.

Pregnancy

If mating is with a fertile male, fertilisation takes place in the uterine tubes (also called the Fallopian tube or oviduct). The early embryo passes into the uterine horn after 4–5 days and implantation occurs after 12–16 days. Prior to implantation the embryos move along the uterine horns so that they are evenly distributed in both. The gestation period is 64 days from the first mating and during this time the corpora lutea remain the sole source of *progesterone*, which is elevated until the precipitous drop at parturition.

From about day 20–30 the placenta begins to produce *relaxin*. Relaxin may act to support the corpus luteum during pregnancy (since the corpus luteum of a non-pregnant animal regresses earlier than the corpus luteum of pregnancy) either by acting on the corpus luteum directly or by acting on the anterior pituitary to produce prolactin.

Prolactin levels increase around day 25–35 of pregnancy (just when relaxin levels are rising) and are maximal just before parturition. Prolactin helps to maintain the corpus luteum in cats and is therefore *luteotropic*.

Pregnancy diagnosis

It is usually fairly easy to determine pregnancy in the cat simply by abdominal palpation at 3–4 weeks and after 6–7 weeks of gestation. Confirmation of pregnancy can be achieved using transabdominal ultrasonography. It is also possible to measure relaxin levels in the blood since this is a pregnancy specific hormone but in practice this is rarely done.

Parturition

Parturition is divided into three stages:

- *First stage labour* is the onset of increased uterine contractions. It usually lasts for 6–12 hours but may be as long as 36 hours. During this time the vagina and cervix relax but there is no abdominal straining. The queen will appear restless and uncomfortable. The pre-parturient drop in rectal temperature is not so obvious in the cat as it is in the bitch. The progesterone decline is first brought about by converting it to oestrogen. This conversion is triggered by corticosteroids from the fetus. Once progesterone levels drop and oestrogen levels rise, the myometrial contractions increase and the cascade of events take place that result in parturition (see physiology of parturition).
- *Second stage labour* begins when abdominal straining starts. The abdominal straining results in the engagement of the fetus in the pelvic canal. At this stage the chorioallantoic membrane may rupture. If so, there is an expulsion of chorioallantoic fluid. This fluid has a reddish-brown colour, which comes from the pigmentation at the edge of the zonary placenta. The fetus is expelled through the pelvic canal still within the amniotic membrane. The queen normally breaks the membrane and then cleans the newborn (neonate) with vigorous licking. She also bites through the umbilical cord. The first kitten is usually expelled within an hour of second stage labour beginning.
- *Third stage labour* is the expulsion of the fetal membranes (placenta). Usually each membrane

follows the fetus within about 15 minutes. However, it is not uncommon for two or three fetuses to be born before the placentae appear. The queen will often eat the placentae. This can cause vomiting and diarrhoea.

In general it is best to leave the queen to kitten in peace. However, occasionally it is necessary to intervene to help. Intervention in the parturient queen is similar to that in the bitch.

Nursing assistance at parturition

- Sometimes the amniotic membrane does not break easily. It is important that this is not delayed because the kitten needs to gain oxygen via the lungs once the placental exchange of oxygen has been compromised. The attending nurse may need to break the amniotic membrane if the queen does not do so.
- Sometimes the fetal airways are blocked with fetal fluids or mucus. The airways need to be cleared and obstructions removed to allow normal breathing. This can be achieved either by gentle suction with a plastic pipette or by swinging the fetus to allow gravity and centrifugal forces to act. *This latter procedure must be carried out with great care* – over-enthusiastic swinging will cause cranial haemorrhage and can kill the newborn kitten.
- The umbilicus may need to be cut. Usually the queen will bite the cord to break it but if not it can be clamped with sterile forceps and cut with sterile scissors. If the forceps are left on for about 10 minutes there may be no need to ligate. If there is haemorrhage then an absorbable ligature should be applied. Approximately 2cm of umbilical cord should be left attached to the kitten. Cutting the cord too close to the ventral abdominal wall may result in a hernia.

Parturition is usually completed within 6 hours of the onset of second stage labour and should not be allowed to continue for more than 24 hours.

THE TOM

The male cat (tom) is sexually active the whole year round.

Puberty is defined as when the cat starts to produce spermatozoa in the ejaculate. It occurs on average about 1–2 months later than females, at 8–12 months old. It can vary with breed and be as late as 18 months old or as early as 7 months. At the onset of puberty the penis begins to develop cornified papillae. These papillae are androgen dependent and develop as testosterone levels begin to rise.

Normal testes

The testes are descended into the scrotum at birth but can be retracted into the inguinal ring at will until about 4–6 months old. Spermatogenesis in the tom is similar to that in the dog.

Cryptorchidism and cryptorchids

Failure of the testes to descend into the scrotum is called *cryptorchidism* and the animal is said to be a cryptorchid. Failure of only one testis to descend is *unilateral* cryptorchidism. Unilateral cryptorchids can be fertile because the descended testis will produce spermatozoa. There is a possible breed disposition for cryptorchidism in Persian cats.

Accessory glands of the tom cat

Cats have a prostate located at the neck of the bladder and bulbourethral glands caudal to the prostate. Both the prostate and the bulbourethral glands are androgen dependent.

Mating

Once the tom mounts the female (see above) intromission and ejaculation is very rapid, just a few seconds. The ejaculate is not fractionated as in the dog and is of very small volume; just one or two drops (Box 11.2).

Secondary sex characteristics

The secondary sex characteristics are those induced by the effects of testosterone. In the tom cat these are:

- the thickened skin on the cheek pouches and scruff of the neck caused by increased subcutaneous connective tissue

> **Box 11.2 Normal ejaculate characteristics in the tom cat**
>
> - Volume: 0.01–0.77ml
> - % motile sperm*: 60–95%
> - % morphologically normal sperm: >60%
> - Number of sperm per ejaculate*: $3–153 \times 10^6$
>
> *Parameter very variable

- the more muscular appearance of the male due to the anabolic steroid effects of testosterone
- the typical 'tommy odour' of the tom cat.

MANIPULATION OF REPRODUCTION IN THE CAT

The principles of manipulation of reproduction in the queen are similar to those in the bitch. Manipulation of reproduction in the cat is less common than in the dog.

Induction of cyclicity

Cats that are kept in colonies are usually kept on a constant day light length of 16 hours. This amount of light stops the winter anoestrus by stopping the melatonin from suppressing the hypothalamus. Thus the queens will come into season throughout the year.

Induction of ovulation

The queen is an induced ovulator. Ovulation is induced by stimulation of neural receptors on the back and within the vagina. Thus ovulation can be induced by stimulating the vagina and stroking the queen when she is in oestrus. This will cause an LH surge and induce ovulation. This procedure is only effective if the queen has already produced follicles. It is used to stop queens calling when the owners do not want them to breed. After ovulation the queen has 30–45 days of pseudopregnancy.

Suppression of oestrus

In the queen this can be achieved either by inducing endogenous progesterone secretion or by providing exogenous progesterone.

- Endogenous progesterone can be produced by inducing ovulation as above and therefore producing corpora lutea. The corpora lutea will produce *progesterone* and this will stop the oestrous behaviour – which is dependent on oestrogen. Ovulation and the production of corpora lutea will also delay the return to oestrus, which, in the absence of ovulation, occurs every three weeks.

- Exogenous progesterone can be provided in a similar manner as in the bitch, i.e. in tablet form or by injection. Progesterone inhibits GnRH release and so the queen will not return to oestrus until the administration of progesterone is stopped.

Castration

As in the dog, castration not only removes the source of sperm but also the source of *testosterone*.

12

Reproductive physiology of the horse

Core information: **The mare is seasonally polyoestrus and oestrus is induced by increased day length. During pregnancy cells from the embryonic membranes migrate into the endometrium of the mare to produce the endometrial cups. Endometrial cups produce equine chorionic gonadotropin (eCG), which stimulates production of accessory corpora lutea. The endometrial cups have a life span that is not reduced if the embryo dies. Hence, if the embryo does die the mare cannot return to oestrus until the endometrial cups regress. Pregnancy is maintained by progesterone produced first of all from the corpus luteum of ovulation, then the corpora lutea induced by the endometrial cups, and lastly from the placenta. The mare is unusual in that there are high levels of circulating oestrogen in the middle third of pregnancy.**

THE MARE

The mare is a seasonal breeder. The hypothalamus begins to secrete gonadotropin releasing hormones (GnRH) in response to an increase in daylight length. Once the mare starts to cycle she will continue until day length begins to decrease in the autumn. Thus she is described as seasonally polyoestrus. The natural breeding season is from approximately May until about October, after which the mare goes into anoestrus.

Puberty

Puberty occurs between 12 and 24 months old and depends upon the time of year the animal is born, nutrition and climate/temperature. However, fillies are not usually bred until they are at least 3 years old.

The oestrous cycle

The natural breeding season in the mare is the spring and summer. During late autumn and winter the mare is in anoestrus. The transition between anoestrus and cyclic activity in the spring is characterised by irregular follicular development and regression. This may continue for a number of weeks and is called the *spring transitional period*. Hormonally the spring transitional period is characterised by low progesterone levels, increasing GnRH release and increasing levels of luteinising hormone (LH).

Eventually a follicle develops and ovulates and then the mare continues to cycle. The cycle length, i.e. the interval between one ovulation and the next, is 19–22 days. As the autumn progresses the mare is less and less likely to produce a follicle and she slips into anoestrus. The period between the end of the breeding season and winter anoestrus is called the *autumn transitional phase*. At this time mares may have a persistent corpus luteum or luteinisation of a follicle. Sometimes mares just have the reverse of the spring transitional phase.

The oestrous cycle can be divided into oestrus, when the mare accepts the stallion and the dominant hormone is oestrogen, and the luteal phase, which is the period after ovulation when the dominant hormone is progesterone.

Oestrus

This is the period when the mare is receptive to the stallion. It can be variable in length and last from as little as 2 days to as long as 12 days, but is more commonly 5–6 days. Oestrus is shorter during the peak of the breeding season and relates to the time needed for the ovulatory follicle to develop. During oestrus the follicles are growing and producing oestrogen – the hormone responsible for making the mare receptive to the stallion.

Early in the oestrous period the mare has a number of follicles that are roughly the same size but eventually one follicle, the dominant follicle, enlarges and this is the one that will ovulate. Between 24–48 hours after ovulation the mare is no longer receptive to the male. Ovulation is due to an LH surge from the anterior pituitary, triggered by the rising oestrogen levels. Receptivity to the male is lost because after ovulation the oestrogen levels fall and progesterone levels begin to rise.

The mare usually produces only one follicle that ovulates, but some mares have a tendency to have double ovulations. The incidence of twin ovula-tions is higher in the spring transitional period and can range from 4% to 44% of ovulations. The average number of twin ovulations is approximately 16%. However, twin conceptions are rarely carried to term.

Oestrous behaviour

When the mare is receptive, if she is presented to the stallion she will allow him to approach her. She will squat, lift the tail and open and close the vulval lips (a behaviour called 'winking') and squirt drops of urine. This will encourage the stallion and the mare will stand to allow mounting. (If she is not receptive she will kick out when the stallion approaches.)

Luteal phase

This is often called dioestrus, the time when the corpus luteum develops from the ruptured follicle. After ovulation the ruptured follicle fills with a blood clot – this is called the corpus haemorrhagicum. Luteal cells grow into the clot and the body becomes the corpus luteum. The dominant hormone at this stage is progesterone. Progesterone suppresses GnRH release so that although follicles are present in the ovary in this phase, they regress before getting large enough to ovulate. The corpus luteum secretes progesterone for 14–15 days, then it regresses. Regression of the corpus luteum is caused by prostaglandin $F_{2\alpha}$, which is produced by the endometrium after progesterone priming. The drop in progesterone removes the block to GnRH secretion, the follicles grow bigger and the mare comes back into oestrus.

Occasionally the corpus luteum fails to regress. The reason for this is not always known. The failure of regression produces a prolonged luteal phase and could be mistaken for pregnancy by some owners.

Pregnancy

The physiology of pregnancy in the mare is very unusual. The pregnancy is maintained by progesterone but the source of progesterone varies as gestation progresses. Gestation length is approximately 11 months (335–342 days) but can vary greatly. There is some evidence that day length will affect gestation length in that mares foaling in winter or early spring tend to have gestation lengths about 10 days longer than mares foaling in the summer. In addition, male foals tend to be carried 2–3 days longer than female foals.

After ovulation the corpus luteum produces progesterone. Normal regression of the corpus luteum has to be inhibited by the conceptus in order for pregnancy to be maintained. The exact mechanism for fetal recognition in the mare is not understood but it does require the early conceptus to move around the uterus and touch the endometrial lining in a number of places. In some way, this inhibits the production of prostaglandin and therefore the corpus luteum of pregnancy (primary corpus luteum) is retained.

After implantation, which occurs around day 15–16, some fetal embryonic cells migrate into the maternal uterine tissue and form groups of secretory cells called endometrial cups. At 35–40 days after fertilisation the endometrial cups secrete equine chorionic gonadotropin (eCG) (eCG was also known as pregnant mare serum gonadotropin – PMSG). eCG is luteotropic (i.e. sustains the corpus luteum) – it has a number of actions:

- maintenance of the primary corpus luteum
- induction of ovulation and/or luteinisation of other ovarian follicles so that they form secondary corpora lutea which also produce progesterone.

The level of eCG depends upon parity, the number of embryos and the genotype of the fetus, the sire and the dam. Ponies tend to have higher levels of eCG than larger horses. Peak concentrations of eCG are at about 60 days of gestation.

After the establishment of the endometrial cups they still continue to function even if the embryo dies. Therefore, if the embryo dies after the endometrial cups are formed the mare does not come back into season again until the endometrial cups have regressed.

By about 100–120 days the production of eCG stops, and by about 130-180 days the endometrial cups are fully rejected by the maternal endometrium. Thus, by about 200 days all the corpora lutea have regressed and so they are no longer the source of progesterone. However, from about day 30–70 the placenta produces progesterone, which supports the pregnancy once the corpora lutea have regressed (Fig.12.1). The progesterone produced by the placenta acts locally and so peripheral blood levels of progesterone appear low.

The mare is unusual in that the placenta produces high levels of oestrogens during the middle third of pregnancy (Box 12.1). The high levels of oestrogens result in the fetal gonads (both male and female) becoming greatly enlarged between the third and ninth month of gestation. At their height a female fetus can have ovaries larger than the dam's. After about day 250 the fetal gonads regress in size and at birth they are only about one-tenth of their fetal size.

Relaxin is also produced by the placenta and levels increase from about day 70 onwards. Levels plateau by about the 5th month of gestation and then increase again just before parturition.

Pregnancy diagnosis

Early pregnancy diagnosis in the thoroughbred mare is particularly important because of the problems of twin conceptions. Twin pregnancies

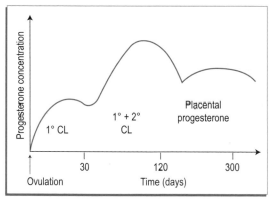

Figure 12.1 Diagrammatic representation of sources and levels of progesterone during pregnancy in the mare.

Box 12.1 Placental oestrogens in the mare

From about 60 days of pregnancy the placenta starts to produce oestrogenic compounds, which are excreted in the urine. The main oestrogens are oestrone, equilin and equilenin.

are usually not carried to term but are lost after the establishment of the endometrial cups. Thus, unless the twins are diagnosed and aborted before 42 days it will not be possible to re-serve the mare early enough in the season. There are a number of methods available for pregnancy diagnosis in the mare:

- *Per rectum uterine palpation.* At 15–18 days after service there is an increase in uterine tone in the pregnant animal compared to the non-pregnant. From 20 days onwards the embryonic vesicle can be palpated to one side or other of the T junction of the uterine horns. Between 60–100 days palpation is difficult and from 3–4 months onwards the fetus can again be felt.
- *Per rectum real time ultrasonography.* From 18 days onwards the embryonic vesicle can be visualised by per rectum ultrasonography. This is the principle method of pregnancy diagnosis used in thoroughbred studs.
- *Equine chorionic gonadotropins (eCG).* Between 40 and 120 days the endometrial cups are secreting eCG, which can be detected in the blood. However, this test can give a false positive because the endometrial cups will continue secreting even although the embryo has died.
- *Oestrone sulphate.* After 60 days the oestrone sulphate secreted by the placenta will be detectable in the blood. Since oestrone sulphate is only produced by a viable placenta this test does not give false positives.
- *Urinary oestrogens.* The raised blood oestrogens are secreted via the urine and so urinary oestrogens can be used for pregnancy diagnosis.

Parturition

The gestation period in the mare is approximately 11 months. The hormone levels in the peripar-turient mare are different from those of other domestic animals and the onset of parturition is poorly understood. Progesterone levels rise towards the last 30 days of gestation and then fall pre-cipitously just prior to parturition. Oestrogen levels start to decline after about 300 days of gestation.

The udder begins to enlarge as early as 3–4 weeks before parturition but the major growth is in the last two weeks of pregnancy. Approximately 1–2 days before the onset of parturition the teats develop a waxy plug, which indicated the presence of colostrum.

First stage labour
This is the period of increased uterine contractions and the mare will sweat, be restless and keep lying down and getting up. She may urinate and look at her flanks. During this period the fetus is rotating to assume the correct posture for delivery.

Second stage labour
This is when voluntary abdominal straining starts. The cervix opens and the chorioallantoic membrane protrudes into the vagina. Usually the mare is lying down on her side (i.e. she is in lateral recumbency) at this stage. The chorioallantoic membranes break and the chorioallantoic fluids are expelled. This reveals the amnion (the membrane surrounding the foal) and the foal's front feet with the nose between. The foal should be delivered within 30 minutes of these 'waters' breaking.

Final expulsion is rapid and due to violent abdominal straining. The foal is delivered still within the amniotic membrane, which breaks as the front feet are pushed through when the foal attempts to stand. The normal presentation and position for the foal is the two front feet extended and the head extended between them.

Once the head and shoulders of the foal are delivered the mare rests, still lying down and still with the foal's hind legs in the vagina. This is an important period during which placental blood is draining back into the foal. If the mare gets up too soon the umbilicus is broken and the foal may fail to gather a significant volume of blood.

The mare has a certain amount of voluntary control over the start of second stage labour. Approximately 70% of mares foal at night between 10pm and 2am. This may be a mechanism to allow her to foal in the peace and quiet. Hence many mares are monitored remotely by cameras so that intervention can be rapid if necessary but the mare feels secure.

Third stage labour
This is the delivery of the fetal membranes, i.e. the placenta, which should occur by about 1 hour after

the birth of the foal – and certainly within 3–4 hours. Failure to expel the fetal membranes can lead to serious illness and needs veterinary attention.

Post-partum return to oestrus

After parturition mares can return to oestrous activity very quickly. The first oestrus occurs in approximately 9 days and is called the *foal heat*. If the mare has a foal-at-foot oestrus can be suppressed by suckling. This is because prolactin suppresses GnRH and so blocks cyclic activity.

THE STALLION

The testes descend into the scrotum within the last three weeks of pregnancy or the first two weeks of life.

Puberty

Puberty occurs at about 18–24 months old but is very variable – it depends on the time of year when born, nutrition and breed. The testes are not fully mature until the stallion is about 5–7 years old.

Accessory glands

The stallion has four sets of accessory glands:

- The ampullae, which are the dilated ends of the ductus deferens. They secrete fluid and also store sperm.
- The prostate gland. Prostatic secretions are watery in nature and are part of the sperm-rich fraction of the ejaculate.
- Seminal vesicles. Secretion from these glands is quite gelatinous and forms the gel fraction of the ejaculate.
- Bulbourethral glands. These produce the pre-sperm fraction of the ejaculate.

Accessory glands produce most of the fluid of the ejaculate. They support the sperm and help to carry the sperm into the uterus.

The ejaculate can be divided into three fractions, pre-sperm fraction, sperm-rich fraction and gel fraction. The volume of ejaculate in the stallion is quite large, ranging from 50ml to >100ml when the gel fraction is included (Box 12.2).

All the accessory glands are testosterone dependent and reduce in size after castration, although this is less noticeable for the bulbourethral glands.

Mating behaviour

The stallion approaches towards the head of the mare first and will snicker and nibble at the neck. He will sniff the urine that the mare in season will produce and then show 'flehmen'. This is a characteristic male behaviour and involves the stallion lifting his head, curling the upper lip and sucking in air. During this time the penis is partially erect and protruded.

He will mount the mare by locking his forelegs over the pelvic bone and often he will bite the neck of the mare as if to hold her. In supervised matings the mare often wears a thick neck cape to protect her from injury and she has boots on the hind feet to protect the stallion should she kick out.

When intromission is achieved ejaculation takes place over a period of a few minutes. During this time the tail of the stallion is lifted up and down (this is called flagging) in time with pulsatile contractions of the pelvic muscles. There are also pulsatile contractions along the penis. In supervised matings the groom will often place a hand on the shaft of the penis so that he can detect these contractions and ensure that the stallion is actually ejaculating.

After ejaculation the stallion dismounts and the erection is lost. Some stallions dismount without having ejaculated but in this instance the erection is usually maintained.

Box 12.2 Normal ejaculate characteristics of the stallion

- Volume*: 60–70ml
- % motile sperm: >50%
- % morphologically normal sperm†: >50%
- Number of sperm per ejaculate: $4–14 \times 10^9$

*In addition, there will be a gel fraction that is usually filtered off before ejaculate evaluation.
†Parameter very variable.

Cryptorchidism

Horses in which the testes have remained within the abdomen are known as 'rigs'. There can be unilateral rigs (one retained testis) or bilateral rigs (both testes retained in the abdomen). Rigs will show male behaviour because testosterone is still produced by the Leydig cells. Undiagnosed rigs can be a problem to handle and difficult to ride. It is possible to check to see if there is an abdominal testis.

Diagnosis of a rig

There are two physiological tests available to diagnose a retained testis.

- *The hCG challenge test.* hCG is human chorionic gonadotropin and has LH-like activity. A rig will respond to the injection of hCG by producing a peak of testosterone secreted by the Leydig cells in the retained testis. The test is carried out by taking a blood sample before the hCG challenge to establish basal levels of testosterone. The suspect rig is then injected with hCG and 30 minutes later a second blood sample is taken to see if the testosterone levels have risen. This test can be used to diagnose a cryptorchid male of any species.
- *Oestrone sulphate test.* The stallion is unusual in that the testis produces high levels of oestrone sulphate (oestrone sulphate is not a biologically active oestrogen and so does not affect the 'maleness' of the stallion). In horses over 3 years of age a single blood sample can be taken and the oestrone sulphate levels measured. A cryptorchid animal will have high levels of oestrone sulphate. This test is not suitable for horses younger than 3 years, or other species of any age, not even donkeys.

MANIPULATION OF REPRODUCTION

Manipulation of the breeding season is most common in thoroughbred studs. This is because thoroughbreds are all aged for racing purposes as if they were born on the 1st of January. Therefore the nearer to the 1st of January the actual birth occurs the greater the advantage the animal has.

Induction of early cyclicity

This is achieved by providing extra artificial light from the beginning of December. This reduces melatonin secretion and releases this hormone's block on GnRH. Increased secretion of GnRH results in increased levels of follicle stimulation hormone (FSH) and follicular development. At least 16 hours of light must be provided in the stable and the brightness is usually quoted as being 'sufficient to read a newspaper'.

Shortening the spring transitional period

It is possible to reduce the time between the onset of follicular growth (i.e. the start of the spring transitional period) and the eventual growth and ovulation of a mature follicle by the administration of exogenous progesterone orally in the food. The progesterone is given for 10–16 days and then withdrawn. The effect is as if the animal had had its own corpus luteum producing progesterone. When the exogenous progesterone is withdrawn there is a rebound rise in GnRH, which produces FSH – this triggers follicular maturation with an oestrogen rise, followed by an LH surge and ovulation.

Shortening the luteal phase

The corpus luteum can be made to regress by the administration of exogenous prostaglandin between days 5–12 after oestrus. This is sometimes done for:

- clinical reasons if there is a uterine infection
- if a mare fails to hold to a service and owners want to reserve her quickly
- to abort a twin pregnancy before the endometrial cups are established at 35 days of pregnancy.

Further reading

- Bowling A T 1996 Horse genetics. CABI Publishing, New York
- Feldman E C, Nelson R W 2004 Canine and feline endocrinology and reproduction, 3rd edn. W B Saunders, Philadelphia
- Gough A, Thomas A 2004 Breed disposition to disease in dogs and cats. Blackwell Publishing, Oxford
- Nicholas F W 2003 Introduction to veterinary genetics, 2nd edn. Blackwell Publishing, Oxford
- Robinson R 1990 Genetics for dog breeders, 2nd edn. Pergamon Press, Oxford
- Ruvinsky A, Sampson J 2001 The genetics of the dog. CABI Publishing, New York
- Simpson G, England G, Harvey M (eds) 1998 Manual of small animal reproduction and neonatology. BSAVA, Gloucester
- Vella C et al 1999 Robinson's Genetics for cat breeders and veterinarians, 4th edn. Pergamon Press, Oxford

Glossary

Acrocentric This refers to the position of the centromere on the chromosome and means that the centromere is at or very near one end of the chromosome.

Alleles Alternative form of genes.

Aneuploid Refers to cells or individuals having one or just a few whole chromosomes more or less than the diploid number.

Aneuploidy Having one more or less than the normal number of chromosomes.

Autosome Any chromosome that is not a sex chromosome.

Autosomal genes Genes located on chromosomes other than the sex chromosomes.

Backcross The crossing of the F_1 offspring with either of the parents.

Barr body The sex chromatin.

Bivalent A pairing configuration of homologous chromosomes during meiosis.

Cell cycle The life cycle of the cell.

Centromere The region on the chromosome where spindle fibres attach during mitosis or meiosis.

Chiasma The point of attachment between chromatids of two homologous chromosomes during meiosis where exchange can take place.

Chromatid The longitudinal units of a chromosome after DNA synthesis but before centromere separation. One of two new chromosomes after DNA synthesis before centromeric division.

Collateral relatives Relatives which are not ancestors or descendants.

Correlation A measure of how two traits tend to move together. Statistically it may vary from −1.00 to +1.00.

Crossing over The exchange of parts of homologous chromosomes during synapsis of meiosis.

Cytogenetics The study of chromosomes.

Cytokinesis Cytoplasmic division.

Deletion A structural change in chromosomes resulting in the loss of genetic material.

Diploid Normal number of chromosomes in a cell. Since chromosomes come in pairs the diploid number is $2n$ where n is the haploid number of chromosomes.

Diplotene Stage of meiotic prophase during which chromatids start to separate.

Dizygotic twins Twins derived from two separate fertilised eggs. They are no more alike than full brothers or sisters.

Dominant Describes a gene that covers up the expression of its allele when paired together in a cell.

Eplstasis Interaction of two or more pairs of genes that are not alleles.

Euchromatin That part of the chromosome that is pale staining and contains most of the coding areas (genes).

Eukaryotic Refers to plants and animals that have cells with a nucleus with a nuclear membrane and chromosomes which divide by mitosis and meiosis.

Euploid Individuals with the normal chromosome complement.

F_1 generation The first filial generation following the parental, or P_1, generation.

F_2 generation The second filial generation following the parental generation.

Freemartin A sterile female twin to a male.

Gamete Mature ovum or spermatozoon.

Gene Specific sequence of DNA which codes for a sequence of amino acids.

Gene locus The position along the chromosome where the gene is located.

Gene mutation A change in the gene structure.

Generation interval The average age of the parents when the offspring are first born.

Genotype The genetic make-up of an individual as determined by its genes.

Germ cell A gamete or one of the immature precursors.

Gonad The ovary in the female and the testis in the male.

Gonadotropins Hormones released by gonadotroph cells in the anterior pituitary; i.e. follicle stimulating hormone (FSH) and luteinising hormone (LH).

Half-sib Half-brother or half-sister.

Haploid The number of chromosomes in the gamete. Half the diploid number of chromosomes. Denoted as *n*.

Heritability This is the proportion of the variation in the phenotype of a population that is due to a variation in the genotype.

Heterosis Hybrid vigour. The superiority of the heterozygous offspring over the parents.

Heterozygote An individual which possesses unlike alleles.

Homozygote An individual which possesses like alleles.

Hybrid The progeny of parents that are genetically unlike.

Hybrid vigour Heterosis.

Inbreeding The production of offspring by parents more closely related than the average of the population.

Intersex An individual with gonads and/or sex characteristics of both sexes. Usually sterile.

Karyotype The chromosome number and morphology of an individual.

Line breeding A form of inbreeding in which an attempt is made to concentrate the genes of one ancestor or line of ancestors.

Linkage Two or more genes located on the same chromosome so that they tend to be transmitted together.

Linkage group Group of genes located on the same chromosome.

Locus The region on the chromosome where a particular gene is located.

Mendel's 1st Law Alleles separate to different gametes.

Mendel's 2nd Law There is independent assortment of non-homologous chromosomes.

Mixaploid An individual with a mixed population of cells relative to their chromosome complement.

Mutation A change in the sequence of base pairs in the DNA molecule.

Nicking The production of progeny that are superior to the parents. Similar to heterosis.

Nucleosome A core of histone proteins with two coils of DNA.

Opisthotonus A spasm of the body with the head and back bowed backwards.

Overdominance The interaction of pairs of genes to produce a phenotypic effect that is superior in the heterozygote compared to either homozygote.

Outcross The mating of one individual to another not closely related.

Partial dominance A gene which is only partially dominant to its own allele.

Penetrance The percentage of times a gene is expected to be expressed in the phenotype of those carrying it.

Phenotype The appearance or performance of an individual.

Pleiotropy When one gene affects two or more unrelated traits.

Polled A naturally hornless state.

Polygenic inheritance A trait that is determined by many pairs of genes.

Polyploid Refers to a cell which has three (triploid), four (tetraploid) or more complete sets of the haploid number of chromosomes.

Prepotent The ability of a parent to stamp its characteristics on its offspring. Homozygous dominant individuals are prepotent.

Progeny testing The evaluation of the genetic make-up of an individual by the appearance or performance of its progeny.

Prokaryotic Refers to viruses, bacteria and blue-green algae which do not have a membrane-bound nucleus.

Qualitative traits Traits usually determined by a few genes which have a sharp distinction among phenotypes.

Quantitative traits Traits determined by many genes which have no sharp distinction among phenotypes. Environmental factors often greatly affect such traits.

Random mating A system of mating where each male has an equal opportunity of mating with any female in the group.

Recessive gene A gene whose phenotypic expression is masked by its own dominant allele.

Sex chromosomes The pair of chromosomes that carry the sex-determining genes. In mammals these are the X and Y chromosomes.

Sex-limited traits A trait which is limited to expression in one sex only, e.g. milk or egg production.

Sex linkage Refers to the genes that are located on the sex chromosomes. Sometimes more specifically to those genes on the non-homologous portion of the X chromosome and thus sometimes called X-linked genes.

Sibling Offspring from the same parents, i.e. brothers and sisters.

Superfetation Two pregnancies at the same time in the same gestation period in a female.

Telomere The end of a chromosome.

Teratogen A substance that produces congenital malformations in an animal.

-tropin The suffix 'tropin' means to nourish or have an affinity for. Thus, gonadotropins (FSH & LH) stimulate the gonads (ovaries and testes).

Zygote A cell resulting from the union of the male and female gametes.

Units for hormone assay

Hormone concentrations can be cited in international (SI) units or in common units. It is important to be able to distinguish the two and it is useful to be able to convert from one to another.

Hormone	SI unit	Common unit	To convert common to SI unit	To convert SI to common unit
Oestrogen	pmol/L	pg/ml	× 3.67	× 0.273
Progesterone	nmol/L	ng/ml	× 3.18	× 0.315
Prolactin	µg/L	ng/ml	× 1.00	× 1.00
Testosterone	nmol/L	ng/ml	× 3.47	× 0.288

Hereditary eye diseases in the dog covered in the British Veterinary Association/Kennel Club/ International Sheep Dog Society eye scheme

The veterinary nurse is not expected to be familiar with all the inherited eye defects that are covered in the BVA/KC/ISDS scheme. However, the following list is provided as a reference source should any of the conditions be encountered. It is not intended to be exhaustive and specialised ophthalmology texts should be consulted for definitive descriptions.

COLLIE EYE DISEASE OR COLLIE EYE ANOMALY

This is a condition found principally in Collies, as the name implies, but it can be found in other breeds. In Britain it is most common in the Rough and Smooth Collie and the Shetland Sheepdog. It is less common in the Border Collie.

Classically the condition is described as choroidal hypoplasia, i.e. a failure of development of part of the choroid of the eye. It appears as pale patches on the fundus because of lack of retinal and choroidal pigment and tapetum. The choroidal vessels are also abnormal. The condition is best diagnosed when the dog is a puppy because post-natal development of the tapetum can obscure the choroidal hypoplasia in the adult animal.

The condition is congenital (i.e. present at birth) and believed to be caused by a simple autosomal recessive gene with pleiotropic effects.

GENERALISED PROGRESSIVE RETINAL ATROPHY

This condition affects a number of different breeds. As the name suggests the anomaly is progressive and is identifiable at different ages in different breeds of dog (Box A2.1).

Technically the condition is divided into two types but the clinical effect is the same. In one type there is degeneration of the retinal rods and cones and in the second type there is dysplasia (i.e. abnormal development) of the retinal rods and cones. The retinal degeneration results in a progressive loss of sight, which owners first notice when the animal is out at night. Eventually the animal becomes totally blind and a secondary cataract may develop.

The mode of inheritance is a simple autosomal recessive gene – but not the same gene in each breed. The causal gene has been identified in the Irish Setter so that it is now possible to detect heterozygous animals. Identification of carrier animals as well as affected animals would in theory enable the complete eradication of the problem if all animals in the breed were tested.

Box A2.1 Some breeds of dogs in which generalised progressive retinal atrophy is found

Rough Collie
Miniature Long-haired Dachshund
Irish Setter
Elkhound
Miniature and Toy Poodle
Labrador Retriever
Cocker Spaniel and English Springer Spaniel
Welsh Cardigan Corgi
Tibetan Spaniel and Tibetan Terrier

CENTRAL PROGRESSIVE RETINAL ATROPHY

This condition is found in a number of breeds, some of which also have generalised progressive retinal atrophy (Box A2.2).

The disease is caused by a build up of a fatty deposit in retinal pigment cells with a secondary degeneration of the retinal rods and cones. The onset of diagnostic changes in the eye is at a rather older age than in generalised progressive retinal atrophy. Clinically the dogs first present because of an inability to see in bright light whilst coping well in dim conditions (this is almost the opposite of the presentation for generalised retinal atrophy). The condition does not usually progress to total blindness but working dogs cannot work in their normal daylight conditions. It is not usual for a secondary cataract to develop.

The inheritance of central progressive retinal atrophy is complex and may be multifactorial, with poor diet playing a contributory role.

HEREDITARY CATARACT

Cataract is defined as any opacity of the lens or its capsule. There are a number of causes of cataracts and only some cataracts are inherited. Hereditary cataract in the Miniature Schnauzer is congenital and due to an autosomal recessive gene. Other types are not congenital but have an early onset and are progressive (Box A2.3). Most of these are also thought to be caused by an autosomal recessive gene.

PRIMARY LENS LUXATION

This problem is seen in some terrier breeds (Smooth and Wire-haired Fox Terrier, Parson Jack Russell Terrier, Sealyham, Miniature Bull Terrier) and appears when the dogs are about 4 or 5 years old.

When the lens becomes dislocated it is a common cause of secondary glaucoma (see below). It is the glaucoma which causes damage to the optic nerve and blindness. Clinically the presenting signs are pain and lacrimation with a dislike of bright light. The luxated lens must be removed as soon as possible to avoid permanent damage and blindness.

The mode of inheritance is thought to be autosomal recessive in most breeds.

PRIMARY GLAUCOMA

Glaucoma is a persistent elevated pressure in the intraocular fluid. Primary glaucoma is an inherited condition resulting from a defect in the normal drainage and circulation of ocular fluid. There are a number of different anomalies of drainage. There are definite breed and line predispositions but the exact mode of inheritance is not known.

PERSISTENT PUPILLARY MEMBRANE

Normally in the uterus the eye is covered by a membrane that breaks down just before birth. Occasionally the breakdown is incomplete and

---

Box A2.2 Some breeds of dog in which central progressive retinal atrophy is found

Border, Smooth and Rough Collie
Briard
Golden Retriever
Labrador Retriever
Shetland Sheepdog
Cocker Spaniel and English Springer Spaniel
Welsh Cardigan Corgi

Table A2.3 Breeds of dogs with early onset hereditary cataract

Boston Terrier
Cavalier King Charles Spaniel
Miniature Schnauzer
Old English Sheepdog
Staffordshire Bull Terrier
Standard Poodle
Welsh Springer Spaniel

strands remain after birth. This is usually an accidental event. However, in the Basenji such a persistence of the papillary membrane is believed to be genetic in origin. It does not usually cause a problem with sight but if extensive may cause corneal opacity.

PERSISTENT HYPERPLASTIC PRIMARY VITREOUS

This is a condition seen in the Dobermann and Staffordshire Bull Terrier. It appears as a plaque attached to the posterior lens capsule caused by embryonic remnants that have normally regressed soon after birth and retinal dysplasia. Severe lesions can result in marked reduction in sight and even blindness.

The mode of inheritance is believed to be autosomal dominant with variable or incomplete penetrance.

MULTIFOCAL RETINAL DYSPLASIA

This condition manifests as folding of the retina and is seen in the English Springer and American Cocker Spaniel, Cavalier King Charles Spaniel, Golden Retriever and Rottweiler. Because there is only partial retinal detachment most affected dogs can see adequately. However, severely affected animals will have impairment of sight.

TOTAL RETINAL DYSPLASIA

In this condition the retina is completely detached and therefore the affected animal is totally blind. It is seen in Bedlington Terriers, Labrador Retrievers and Sealyham Terriers. Retinal dysplasia is believed to be caused by a simple autosomal recessive gene.

Appendix 3

Coat colour genetics

Coat colour genetics is quite a complex subject. Nevertheless there are a few coat colour patterns that are sufficiently common to be of interest in a book of this nature.

In mammals the coat colour pattern is derived from melanins in the skin and hair. Melanins are found in specialised cells called melanocytes. There are two types of melanins: eumelanin and pheomelanin. Eumelanin will produce a black colour which can be modified to produce blue-black or chocolate-brown which is often called 'liver' by dog breeders. Pheomelanin will produce a reddish-brown or yellowish-tan colour in dogs. White, i.e. an absence of colour, is produced either by an absence of melanocytes or by a suppression of their production of pigment.

Variation in coat colour is produced by genes that control the switch between the production of the two types of melanin and/or the presence and arrangement of the pigment granules. There are a number of different genes that control coat colour and many of these genes have alleles. A completely different set of genes control the hair structure. Thus hair can be long or short, wiry or smooth, wavy or curled.

COAT COLOUR GENETICS IN THE DOG

A few of the more important coat colour genes in the dog are discussed below.

1. *Agouti series.* This series controls the distribution of eumelanin and hence the black colour. The agouti A allele allows little eumelanin on the body and produces the wolf grey colour. The A^s allele produces a solid colour over the whole body; the actual colour depends on other coat colour genes. The A^y allele produces hair which is mainly pheomelanin (yellowish) with eumelanin (black) tips. The original name for this allele was dominant yellow but when there are marked black tips the fur has a sable colour and so this allele is also called sable. Another allele is a^t, which is recessive to the other two and produces a black-and-tan pattern. The body is eumelanic (black) with pheomelanic (yellow or tan) patches over the eyes, on the muzzle, chest, belly and around the anus. An example of this colouration is seen in Dobermanns. The non-agouti allele, a, is recessive and produces a black colour because eumelanin is produced.

2. *The extension alleles.* These alleles control the proportion of eumelanin and pheomelanin. The most common allele is designated E and is the normal extension gene and extends the amount of eumelanin and thus produces a black colour. Within this series there is a recessive allele, e, which diminishes the amount of eumelanin and increases the amount of pheomelanin thus producing a yellow coat colour. A third allele E^{br} is dominant to E and produces stripes of black over yellow which is the brindle effect. Extension alleles interact with agouti alleles.

3. *Black and brown alleles.* The colour black is produced by the dominant B allele which makes black eumelanin and the pigments granules are oval and intense. The recessive b allele produces brown eumelanin and smaller and rounded granules which appears to change the colour to our (human) eyes to brown.

4. *The Merle gene.* There is a dominant gene, M, which causes a white coat in the homozygous state. There are other effects such as abnormally

small eyes with blue irises, partial or complete deafness and sometimes sterility. The normal allele, *m*, is recessive and allows normal colour distribution. The homozygous animal, *Mm*, produces a pale coat with dapples of darker areas classically seen in, for example, rough and smooth collie dogs.

5. *Dilution gene.* All white dogs can be the result of a recessive dilution gene *d* which reduces the number of pigment granules in the hair so that there appears to be no colour.

6. *White spotting.* Some white dogs can be the result of the recessive white spotting gene, *s*, which produces patches of white in the coat and in extreme conditions the 'patch' of white extends over the whole body.

7. *Albino alleles.* A third way to produce a white dog is via the recessive albino gene, *c*. The homozygous dog will be white with pink eyes. Another allele in the series, c^b produces an albino dog with blue irises. Dogs with the normal coat colour have the dominant normal colour gene, *C*.

The most common questions asked concerning coat colour genetics in the dog relate to the Labrador Retriever which can be black, brown (also called liver) and yellow. Yellow Labradors can have either a black nose or brown/liver nose. The different colours in the Labrador retriever are easily explained with reference to the three main gene series: agouti, extension and black/brown.

Black Labrador Retrievers

These animals are black all over and therefore must have the dominant A^S (solid) allele in the agouti series. They are 'black' and therefore must have the dominant *B*, black gene, and in order to produce a black colour at all they must be producing eumelanin and therefore must have the dominant E extension allele. Hence the genotype for the black Labrador retriever can be written

$$A^S\text{--},B\text{--},E\text{--}$$

The '–' indicates that it does not matter which other allele is also present at that particular locus. Such an animal will have a black nose.

Brown or Liver Labrador Retrievers

These animals also have the same colour all over and so must have the dominant A^S (solid) allele in the agouti series. However, the brown colour is coded for by the recessive *b* allele which therefore has to be homozygous in order to be expressed. As described above there needs to be eumelanin and so the dominant E extension allele must be present. Thus the genotype for a liver Labrador retriever is written

$$A^S\text{--},bb,E\text{--}$$

Such an animal will have a brown/liver nose.

Yellow Labrador Retrievers with a black nose

The yellow colour is produced by pheomelanin which is coded for by the recessive e extension gene. The black nose needs the dominant *B* gene for black production. The agouti alleles govern the distribution of eumelanin in the hair. Since there is no eumelanin in the hair it does not matter which agouti allele is present. Thus the genotype of the yellow Labrador with a black nose can be written

$$\text{--}\,\text{--},B\text{--},ee.$$

Yellow Labrador Retrievers with a brown/liver nose

In these animals the only difference is that they need to be homozygous for the recessive *b*, brown gene in order to produce the brown nose. Hence the genotype is written

$$\text{--}\,\text{--},bb,ee.$$

COAT COLOUR GENETICS IN THE CAT

The original coat colour in the cat is thought to be the short-coated mackerel striped tabby seen in the European wild cat.

1. *Tabby striping.* There are two main types of tabby pattern. The mackerel-striped tabby has vertical

stripes on the side of the body rather like a tiger. This is produced by the dominant tabby gene, *T*. A second type of tabby pattern is called the blotched tabby. This animal has whirls or blotches of darker colour on the flanks whilst the head and tail markings are similar to those of the mackerel tabby. This pattern is produced by a second allele, *t^b*, which is recessive. A third allele *T^u* produces the coat pattern seen in Abyssinian cats, where the stripes can barely be seen at all.

2. *Non-agouti gene.* The grey colour in the tabby stripes is due to the normal, dominant agouti gene, *A*. This gene has a recessive non-agouti allele, *a*. The animal homozygous for *aa* is all-over black (or another colour if there are other coat colour genes present).

3. *Black/brown alleles.* The dominant gene, *B*, which produces black pigment, has recessive alleles which produce different intensities of brown. A dark chocolate brown is produced by the recessive allele *b* and this is seen in Havana cats. A lighter form (milk chocolate?) is produced by a second recessive allele *b^l*.

4. *Dilution gene.* A recessive gene, *d*, will change black to blue and the dark chocolate colour to lilac. The normal colour is produced in the presence of the dominant, non-dilution gene, *D*.

5. *Dilution modifier.* A dominant gene, *Dm*, lightens further the diluted coat colour but has no effect on the full colour.

6. *Orange gene.* The sex-linked orange gene, *O* has been discussed in chapter 5. It is epistatic to the autosomal coat colour genes and will mask their presence in cells where the X chromosome carrying the orange gene is functional.

7. *White spotting or piebald pattern.* Many cats have some white patches. The extent of spotting varies. There can be just a spot under the chin and on the umbilicus or this can extend to the whole chest and chin and up the flanks. In the most extreme cases the whole of the animal is white. The white spotting gene, *S*, is dominant but the mechanism for producing the variation is not fully understood.

8. *Dominant white.* Another way to produce a completely white cat is via the dominant white gene, *W*. This gene is epistatic to all other coat colour genes. White cats produced by the dominant white gene can have blue eyes or even odd coloured eyes and may be deaf in one or both ears.

9. *Long hair.* Long-haired cats are homozygous for the recessive gene, *l*, whilst short-haired cats have the dominant gene, *L*.

COAT COLOUR GENETICS IN THE HORSE

The major coat colour genes of the horse, i.e. agouti, extension and grey, have been discussed in chapter 2. The production of black, bay and chestnut horses has been described together with greys. It is worth mentioning two other well known colours – white and roan.

1. *The white gene.* There is a dominant gene, *W*, which produces a horse that lacks pigment in the hair and skin from birth (this is unlike greys, which are born with colour that is lost abnormally quickly). Such animals do however, usually have brown eyes. Homozygosity for the white gene is lethal and *WW* foals die in utero.

2. *The dilute gene.* Horses have a dilute gene, *C^cr*, which in the heterozygous state will dilute pheomelanin (which normally produces a brown colour) to a yellow, whilst having no effect on eumelanin. It is therefore incompletely dominant to the normal allele, *C*, which is non-dilute. The homozygous animal, *C^cr C^cr*, will dilute both eumelanin and pheomelanin to produce a white or ivory horse.

3. *The roan gene.* Non-roan, *rn*, is recessive to a dominant mutation, *RN*, which produces a mixing of white hair and coloured hair. Roans are usually *RNrn* since it is believed that homozygosity, *RNRN*, is lethal.

Appendix 4
Miscellaneous abnormalities

In wild populations genetic variations that render animals less fit to cope with life are soon eliminated. Animals carrying the variant gene or genes are either more easily caught by a predator, are less able to find or eat food necessary for their survival, are less attractive to a mate or are less able to reproduce. Conversely, animals carrying a genetic variation that gives them a competitive advantage prosper and their offspring dominate the population. This is the basis of natural selection.

By contrast, as soon as man intervenes and artificially selects for arbitrary attributes then deleterious genetic variation can persist within species or breeds. Whilst each is unlikely to be very common, unless it is in fact a breed requirement, their frequency will be such that the veterinary nurse may encounter them whilst working in practice. The following are a description of some of the anomalies that may be encountered.

CARDIOVASCULAR PROBLEMS

A number of congenital heart problems in dogs have been shown to be inherited, e.g. patent ductus arteriosis (PDA), pulmonic stenosis, aortic stenosis, ventricular septal defect, atrial septal defect, persistent right aortic arch and tetralogy of Fallot. However, because the inheritance of these conditions is multifactorial the degree of disorder is very variable. The situation is similar to the variation in the degree abnormality in hip dysplasia. The same control problems apply to cardiac defects as hip dysplasia – namely the abnormalities are difficult to eliminate, normal animals can produce affected offspring and affected animals can produce normal offspring but are more likely to produce affected offspring.

COMBINED IMMUNODEFICIENCY DISEASE (CID)

This condition is seen in Arabian foals presenting with a very low white cell count and under-developed thymus and lymph nodes. They have a much compromised immune system and die within the first few months of life due to massive infections of any or all of the body systems. The condition is due to an autosomal recessive gene.

CRYPTORCHIDISM

Cryptorchidism is the failure of the testes to descend from the abdomen into the scrotum. Unilateral cryptorchidism is the failure of one testis to descend. Unilateral cryptorchids will be fertile but unilateral cryptorchids are infertile.

The condition is assumed to be inherited in cats, dogs and horses but the mode of inheritance is unknown. It is likely to be polygenic and is the classic example of a sex-limited trait. The condition can only be expressed in the male but the female can also carry the genes that are responsible for the problem.

A unilateral cryptorchid will be fertile but should not be used for breeding and indeed, serious consideration should be given to excluding full sibs, both female as well as male, from the breeding population.

DEAFNESS

Inherited forms of deafness are found in both dogs and cats associated with a white coat colour. This is because a white coat implies an absence of melanocytes and melanocytes are also important in the maintenance of the appropriate environment for the cochlear hair cells in the ear. Lack of melanocytes ultimately results in abnormal cochlear structure and degeneration of the auditory nerve.

In dogs deafness is associated with two different genes. Deafness is associated with homozygosity for the dominant merle gene (*M*). These animals have white coats and blue eyes. As well as being deaf they may also be blind and are infertile. Deafness is also associated with the piebald gene such as that seen in Dalmatians but this does not appear to be a single gene effect. All Dalmatians are homozygous for the recessive piebald gene and this is what gives the breed its characteristic coat colour pattern. Some dogs have an extreme form of piebald caused by the extreme piebald gene (*sw*) and these Dalmatians are exceptionally white. It is these dogs which are likely to be deaf, either unilaterally or bilaterally. Blue-eyed Dalmatians are more likely to be deaf than those with brown eyes. Recent work suggests that the problem is unlikely to be due to a single major gene and that it is likely to be polygenic with threshold expression.

In cats deafness is associated with the autosomal dominant gene for white coat colour (*W*). Such cats have blue irises.

Subjective tests for deafness, such as monitoring the animal's response to sound by ear flicking or turning the head, are unreliable and useless if the animal is unilaterally deaf. An objective measurement of deafness relies on the detection of a response to sound within the brain known as the 'brainstem auditory evoked response' (BAER) using a computer. This test can be carried out in the anaesthetised animals.

Deafness is rarely diagnosed in horses but may be occasionally seen in white horses with the dominant Overo (*O*) spotting gene.

ECTROPION AND ENTROPION

Ectropion is the turning-out of the eyelid and entropion is the turning-in of the eyelid. These conditions can be considered to be inherited only in that the predisposing factors are associated with genetic factors. For example, ectropion is associated with excessive facial skin which allows the lower eyelid to sag, while entropion is associated with the shape of the eye socket. The degree of skin tightness and shape of the eye socket will be controlled by a number of genes.

HAEMOPHILIA A (FACTOR VIII DEFICIENCY)

There are a number of different forms of haemophilia, each resulting in a failure of, or elongation of clotting time of the blood. The different forms of haemophilia are a result of changes in the complex chain of reactions ultimately resulting in the clotting of the blood. Factor VIII is one of the proteins required for blood clotting and its absence results in prolonged bleeding after trauma. Haemophilia A is seen in cats, dogs and horses.

The condition is due to a sex-linked gene, *Hma*, which stops the normal production of factor VIII. Carrier males are affected but carrier females usually have normal or only slightly elongated clotting times because they have a normal gene on the other X chromosome.

HAEMOPHILIA B (FACTOR IX DEFICIENCY)

Haemophilia B is usually more severe in affected animals than haemophilia A. It is seen in cats and dogs and is due to a sex-linked gene, *Hmb*, which is different from the gene causing haemophilia A. This gene causes a deficiency in factor IX, which is another protein necessary in the clotting chain. Other types of haemophilia are shown in Table A4.1.

Table A4.1 **Major defects causing haemophilia**

Type	Heredity	Species
Haemophilia A (Factor VIII deficiency)	Hma – sex-linked	Cats, dogs, horses
Haemophilia B (Factor IX deficiency)	Hmb – sex-linked	Cats and dogs
Factor XII deficiency (Hageman factor)	Hag – incomplete dominant	Cats
Hypofibrinogenaemia (Factor I deficiency)	dominant	Dog
Hypoproconvertinaemia (Factor VII deficiency)	hc – recessive	Dog
Hypothrombinaemia	recessive	Dog
Plasma thromboplastin antecedent (Factor XI deficiency)	pta – dominant	Dog
Stewart–Prower (Factor X deficiency)	stf – dominant	Dog
Thrombasthenia	dominant	Dog
Von Willebrand's disease	Wvd – dominant	Dog

HYPERKALAEMIC PERIODIC PARALYSIS (HYPP)

This is a problem seen in quarter horses. It presents as a generalised muscle tremor, stiffness and paralysis associated with exercise and there is marked elevation of serum potassium levels. The problem is caused by a dominant gene which is a mutant of a normal gene responsible for muscle protein metabolism. Heterozygous animals are usually only mildly affected but homozygous animals will have more problems. A DNA test is available to determine carriers, homozygous and normal animals.

LEGG-CALVE-PERTHE'S DISEASE

This condition is an avascular necrosis of the neck of the femur and presents in young animals of small breeds, e.g. Miniature and Toy Poodles and West Highland White Terriers. In these breeds it is thought to be due to an autosomal recessive gene (*pd*). In Manchester Terriers the results of investigations were more equivocal – in this breed the condition may be polygenic.

PITUITARY DWARFISM

There is a form of dwarfism in the German Shepherd Dog which is due to an autosomal recessive gene (*dw*). The growth retardation begins when the puppy is about two months old.

PANCREATIC INSUFFICIENCY

In the German Shepherd Dog there is one form of pancreatic insufficiency which is caused by an autosomal recessive gene (*pc*). Affected animals are unable to digest food properly and therefore are always very hungry and lose weight despite eating vast amounts of food. The faeces are very characteristic, being copious, pale grey in colour and foul smelling.

PATELLA LUXATION

In this condition the patella moves either medially or laterally out of the groove in the femoral head in which it normally sits. The movement is possible because of mal-development of the femoral groove. It is particularly common in Miniature and Toy Poodles but is seen in other small breeds of dogs. It is also seen with a high incidence in Devon Rex cats.

The condition is inherited but is polygenic with threshold levels of expression. It depends on the development of the femoral groove and patella ligaments.

Congenital lateral patella luxation is also seen in Shetland ponies and in this breed it is thought to be due to a simple autosomal recessive gene.

PROGRESSIVE AXONOPATHY

This is a neurological condition seen in Boxer dogs due to a recessive gene (*pa*). There is degeneration of motor nerve fibres leading to muscular weakness and unco-ordination in movement. Signs are first noted when the affected animal is about 6 months old.

SCOTTIE CRAMP

As the name implies the condition was first seen in Scottish Terriers, but can occur in other breeds, and presents as muscular spasms induced by excitement or strenuous exercise. It is caused by an autosomal recessive gene (*sc*).

UMBILICAL HERNIA

An umbilical hernia indicates a weakness in the umbilical ring. The degree of herniation can be minor, consisting of a small amount of abdominal fat, or can be quite major, with loops of small intestine lying subcutaneously. Narrow faults into which the small intestine can migrate can lead to strangulation and an acute abdominal crisis.

The occurrence of umbilical hernias in both cats and dogs is believed to have a genetic component but the mode of inheritance is not known. It may well be polygenic with threshold levels of expression.

Appendix 5

Questions and answers

This section re-presents some of the material in the book but from a different angle. It is designed to reinforce the student's understanding of the subject matter and therefore facilitate learning. It can be used for individual revision or in a group activity where students can re-enforce the learning of each other. The questions should not be considered to be examples of examination questions and the answers should not be taken as 'model' answers.

Q1. How is the phenotypic sex controlled in mammals?
(a) The presence of a Y chromosome.
(b) The number of X chromosomes.
(c) A cascade of genes throughout the genome.
(d) The male-determining gene.

Answer: (c) Phenotypic sex is controlled by a cascade of genes located throughout the genome. The male-determining gene on the Y chromosome is one in the cascade of genes. Excess X chromosomes, and hence the genes on this chromosome, will inhibit meiosis in the post-pubertal animal.

Q2. How does phenotypic variation arise?
(a) Genetic changes alone.
(b) Environmental changes alone.
(c) Either genetic or environmental changes or both.

Answer: (c) The phenotype can be changed either by changes in genes or changes in the environment or the interaction of the two. The changes can only be passed on to the next generation if there have been genetic changes.

Q3. How do the genes on the pseudo-autosomal segment of the sex chromosomes behave?
(a) Just as the genes on the autosomes.
(b) As sex-linked genes.
(c) As sex-limited genes.

Answer: (a) Genes on the autosomal region of the sex chromosomes act like any other genes located on the autosomes.

Q4. Which of the following statements describes an allele?
(a) One of two or more forms of a gene.
(b) The form of a gene that produces a 'less fit' individual.
(c) The recessive form of the original gene.
(d) The form of the gene that causes an abnormality.

Answer: (a) An allele is a form of a gene produced by a mutation. A succession of mutations will produce an allelic series, i.e. a series of genes all affecting the same characteristic but producing a different result. Some alleles are dominant, some recessive and some co-dominant.

Q5. Which of the following statements describes epistasis?
(a) Epistasis is when more than one gene controls a characteristic.
(b) Epistasis is when one gene on one locus affects the action of another gene on another locus.
(c) Epistasis is when the genes on the X chromosome are switched on.
(d) Epistasis is when the same allele is present at both loci of two homologous chromosomes.

Answer: (b) Epistasis is when one gene affects the action of another gene on another locus. Alleles can affect the action of each other (dominant or recessive) but alleles are at the same locus.

Q6. Sex-limited characteristics are governed by:
   (a) Genes on the X chromosome.
   (b) Genes on the Y chromosome.
   (c) Genes on either the X or Y chromosome.
   (d) Genes on the autosomes.

Answer: (d) Sex-limited characteristics are expressed in only one sex but are governed by genes that are present in both sexes on the autosomes.

Q7. Which of the following statements is *not* correct?
   (a) DNA is made up of a ladder of four different bases.
   (b) DNA consists of chains of functional genes.
   (c) Chromosomes are made up of coiled DNA surrounded by protein.

Answer: (b) DNA is composed of a ladder of bases. The sequence of some of these bases determines the coding function or genes. However, most of the sequences of bases are 'rubbish' DNA and do not code for anything. Therefore DNA cannot be said to be a chain of functional genes alone.

Q8. If a characteristic is governed by a dominant gene how will its expression be shown in a pedigree?
   (a) Every affected individual will have at least one affected parent.
   (b) The mother of an affected individual is always affected.
   (c) All the offspring of an affected individual will be affected.
   (d) All the members of the same litter will be affected.

Answer: (a) Dominant genes will be expressed whenever they are present. Therefore every affected individual will have at least one affected parent but it could be either parent. Affected individuals may only have one copy of the dominant gene and therefore not all the offspring need be affected.

Q9. If a characteristic is governed by a sex-linked dominant gene how will its expression be shown in a pedigree?
   (a) Only females will be affected.
   (b) Only males will be affected.
   (c) Only male offspring of an affected individual will be affected.
   (d) Only female offspring of an affected male will be affected.
   (e) Only female offspring of an affected female will be affected.

Answer: (d) Sex-linked characteristics are governed by genes on the X chromosome. Males are more likely to be affected but females can be affected. Since sex-linked genes are on the X chromosome affected males can only pass the gene to their daughters since their sons receive the Y chromosome. Affected females can pass the X chromosome carrying the sex-linked gene to either their sons or their daughters.

Q10. Which of the following statements is *not* true?
   (a) All intersex dogs are genetic females.
   (b) Some intersex animals are fertile.
   (c) Goats homozygous for the polling gene are intersexes.
   (d) Male tortoiseshell cats are not intersexes.

Answer: (a) An intersex has the external phenotype of one sex and the gonads of the other. This is the situation in goats homozygous for the polling gene, which appears to be linked to an intersexuality gene. Not all intersex dogs are genetic females, although most are. Some hermaphrodite pigs are fertile and male tortoiseshell cats have the phenotype and gonads of males.

Q11. How would you describe the coat colour in tortoiseshell cats?
   (a) Patches of ginger (orange), black and white.
   (b) Patches of ginger (orange) and black.
   (c) Patches of ginger (orange) and non-orange.

Answer: (c) The tortoiseshell coat colour is the expression of the sex-linked orange gene and any another coat colour gene, e.g. black or tabby. The orange gene is epistatic to the other coat colour genes, except white, and so the patches where the orange is expressed must have cells with the X chromosome carrying the orange functional whilst the patches or another colour must have cells with the orange-gene-bearing X chromosome inactivated.

Q12. Which of the following statements is correct?
   (a) It is safe to give an unmatched blood transfusion to a dog.
   (b) Cats do not naturally have antibodies to blood groups different from their own.
   (c) Isoerythrolysis in horses is not a problem in the first foal.

Answer: (c) It is usually safe to give one unmatched transfusion to a dog in an emergency because dogs do not naturally have antibodies to different blood groups before they are challenged. However, subsequent transfusions must be matched. Unlike dogs, cats are like humans and do have antibodies to non-self blood groups. Isoerythrolysis in horses develops after the first foal when the dam and foal have different blood groups and the mare becomes sensitised to the foal's blood group. A second foal with the same blood group will then receive antibodies in the mare's colostrum to its blood.

Q13. Which of the following statements concerning inbreeding are correct?
   (a) Increases homozygosity.
   (b) Reveals recessive genes.
   (c) Depresses fertility.
   (d) Always produces offspring with abnormalities.

Answer: (a), (b) and (c) Inbreeding does not always produce offspring with abnormalities, it depends upon which genes are in the genotype in the first place.

Q14. Which of the following statements concerning cross breeding are correct?
   (a) Cross breeding is better than inbreeding.
   (b) Cross breeding hides recessive genes.

   (c) Cross-bred animals do not carry genes that cause abnormalities.
   (d) Cross-bred animals have hybrid vigour.

Answer: (b) and (d) Cross breeding is not 'better' if what is required is the establishment of homozygosity for genes. Cross-bred animals can carry recessive genes that would cause abnormalities but they are masked because cross-bred animals are heterozygous at more gene loci.

Q15. Which hormone is it most practical to measure in order to determine the best time to mate a bitch?
   (a) Oestrogen.
   (b) Luteinising hormone (LH).
   (c) Progesterone.
   (d) Follicle stimulating hormone (FSH).

Answer: (c) Progesterone begins to rise just before the LH surge and ovulation. Progesterone is easier to measure than LH and so progesterone is the hormone of choice.

Q16. Which hormone is involved with pseudopregnancy in the bitch?
   (a) Progesterone.
   (b) Prolactin.
   (c) Relaxin.
   (d) Oxytocin.

Answer: (b) High prolactin levels produce lactation. This usually occurs at parturition. However, in some non-pregnant bitches progesterone levels fall unusually quickly, triggering prolactin release, or the bitch is over-sensitive to the normal rate of progesterone decline and a prolactin rise is triggered.

Q17. Which methods can be used to suppress oestrus in the bitch?
   (a) Injection of a progestogen.
   (b) Administration of prolactin.
   (c) Ovariectomy.
   (d) Progestogen tablets.

Answer: (a) and (d) Progestogens are compounds which have the same action as progesterone. Progesterone blocks follicle stimulating hormone and follicle development. Follicles secrete oestrogen – the hormone responsible for oestrous behaviour. Ovariectomy is the removal of the ovaries, which is not reversible.

Q18. In the cat what is the consequence of an infertile mating?
   (a) A failure of ovulation.
   (b) Pseudopregnancy.
   (c) Return to oestrus in three weeks.

Answer: (b) Ovulation in the cat is stimulated by coitus. If mating takes place but the tom is infertile, ovulation is still induced and corpora lutea are formed. These secrete progesterone and the cat enters a type of pseudopregnancy.

Q19. What are the endometrial cups in mares?
   (a) The part of the uterus to which the placenta attaches.
   (b) Accessory corpora lutea secreting progesterone.
   (c) Specialised cells of fetal origin.

Answer: (c) The endometrial cups are formed by cells that migrate into the endometrium of the mare from the embryo. They secrete equine chorionic gonadotropin, which stimulates accessory corpora lutea on the ovary.

Q20. Which of the following statements is true?
   (a) Ovulation in the mare occurs at the beginning of behavioural oestrus.
   (b) Ovulation in the bitch occurs at the beginning of behavioural oestrus.
   (c) Ovulation in the cat occurs at the beginning of behavioural oestrus.

Answer: (b) In the mare ovulation occurs after a prolonged period of oestrus behaviour during which the dominant follicle is growing. After ovulation the mare goes out of season. In the cat ovulation is induced by coitus – if no mating takes place there is no ovulation. In the bitch ovulation occurs on about the second day of behavioural oestrus, i.e. when the bitch will allow the dog to mount. She will continue to allow the dog to mount after ovulation and during this time the eggs are maturing and becoming ready to be fertilised.

Q21. Which of the following hormones is secreted by the anterior pituitary in the male?
   (a) Testosterone.
   (b) Luteinising hormone (LH).
   (c) Follicle stimulating hormone (FSH).
   (d) Inhibin.

Answer: (b) and (c) LH and FSH are secreted from the anterior pituitary of the male as well as the female. In the male, LH stimulates the interstitial cells to secrete testosterone and FSH stimulates the Sertoli cells to produce inhibin and androgen binding protein.

Index